Food Revolution

Your Guide To Healthy, Sustainable Eating

A.TEBANI

Table of Contents

Acknowledgement	2
Introduction	3
The Food Revolution Begins	3
Understanding the Basics of Healthy Eating	6
Essential Nutrients and Their Role in Our Body	6
The Importance of Vitamins and Minerals	11
The Power of Whole Foods	13
What Are Whole Foods and Why Do They Matter?	14
How to Transition to a Whole-Food Diet	18
Sustainability Starts on Your Plate	21
Defining Sustainable Eating and Its Global Importance	22
How Food Choices Affect the Planet	24
Understanding Food Miles, Waste, and Resource Use	25
Practical Steps Toward Sustainable Eating	27
The Environmental Impact of Your Diet	30
The Carbon Footprint of Different Food Groups	31
Sustainable Farming and Ethical Sourcing	33
How Plant-Based Diets Contribute to Sustainability	34
Making Sustainable Food Choices	35
Decoding Labels: What You Need to Know	38

How to Read Nutrition Labels and Ingredient Lists	39
Understanding Certifications: Organic, Fair Trade, and Non-GMO	42
Choosing Products with Minimal Environmental Impact	45
Building a Sustainable Pantry	49
Stocking Your Kitchen with Healthy, Eco-Friendly Staples	50
Organic and Local Options for Long-Term Pantry Essentials	53
How to Reduce Food Waste Through Mindful Buying	55
Meal Planning for Health and Sustainability	60
The Importance of Meal Prepping and Planning Ahead	61
How to Create Balanced, Nutritious Meals	63
Sustainable Meal Planning: Reducing Food Waste and Saving Money	66
Navigating Plant-Based Eating	69
The Benefits of a Plant-Based Diet for Health and the Environment	70
How to Get Started with Plant-Based Meals	74
Key Nutrients for Plant-Based Eaters	75
The Role of Meat and Animal Products in a Sustainable Diet	79
The Nutritional Value of Meat and Animal Products	80
The Challenges of Meat and Animal Products	82

How to Incorporate Meat and Animal Products Responsibly	84
Cooking for Health and the Planet	87
Eco-Friendly Kitchen Practices: Energy-Saving Tips and Waste Reduction	88
Healthy Cooking Methods: Steaming, Roasting, and Sauteing	90
How to Create Delicious Meals with a Balance Between Animal and Non-Animal Products	93
Sustainable Eating on a Budget	97
How to Eat Healthily and Sustainably Without Breaking the Bank	98
Cost-Effective Strategies for Sourcing Organic and Local Produce	100
Creative Meal Ideas for Frugal, Nutritious Eating	102
Seasonal Eating: A Guide to Eating with the Seasons	105
The Benefits of Eating In-Season Produce	106
How Seasonal Eating Supports Local Farmers and Reduces Your Carbon Footprint	109
What to Buy Each Season and How to Preserve Excess Produce	110
Reducing Food Waste: Small Steps for Big Change	114
Practical Tips for Reducing Food Waste in the Kitchen	115
Composting: Turning Scraps into Valuable Resources	118

Mindful Consumption: A Shift in Perspective	119
The Bigger Picture: Environmental and Economic Impact	121
The Psychology of Healthy Eating	123
Understanding Food Cravings and Emotional Eating	124
How to Build Healthy, Lasting Habits	126
Staying Committed to Your Sustainable Eating Goals	128
Mindful Eating: Reconnecting with Food	131
The Role of Hydration in Your Diet	140
The Importance of Water for Overall Health	142
The Dangers of Dehydration	142
Sustainable Alternatives to Bottled Water	143
How to Ensure You're Drinking Enough Water Each Day	145
Supplements: Do You Need Them?	149
When and Why to Consider Supplements	151
Sustainable and Natural Supplement Options	153
How to Balance Diet and Supplements for Optimal Health	155
Eating for Long-Term Wellness	159
Building a Diet for Longevity and Disease Prevention	159
Key Lifestyle Habits That Support Lifelong Health	162
The Importance of Variety in Your Diet	163

Conclusion	165
Creating a Sustainable Eating Lifestyle for Your Family	168
How to Make Sustainable Eating Work for All Ages	169
Tips for Encouraging Kids to Eat Healthy, Sustainable Foods	170
Meal Planning and Family-Friendly Sustainable Recipes	172
The Future of Food: Embracing a New Way to Eat	176
Emerging Trends in Sustainable Food Systems	177
The Role of Technology and Innovation in Sustainable Eating	179
Continuing Your Journey Toward a Healthier, More Sustainable Future	181
Conclusion	184
Your Food Revolution Starts Today	184
Resources for Continued Learning	185
Building a Supportive Community for Healthy, Sustainable Eating	188
Your Food Revolution Starts Today	189
References	190

Chapter 1

© Copyright 2025 A.TEBANI 2024 - All rights reserved,

The content within this book may not be reproduced, duplicated or transmitted without direct written permission from the author or the publisher.

Under no circumstances will any blame or legal responsibility be held against the publisher, or author, for any damages, reparation, or monetary loss due to the information contained within this book. Either directly or indirectly. You are responsible for your own choices, actions, and results.

Legal Notice: This book is copyright protected. This book is only for personal use. You cannot amend, distribute, sell, use, quote or paraphrase any part, of the content within this book, without the consent of the author or publisher.

Disclaimer Notice: The information in this document is for education and entertainment only. We have made every effort to provide accurate and current information. We do not guarantee this information in any way. Readers acknowledge that the author is not engaging in the rendering of legal, financial, medical or professional advice. The content within this book has been derived from various sources Please consult a licensed professional before attempting any techniques outlined in this book.

By reading this document, the reader agrees that under no circumstances is the author responsible for any losses, direct or indirect, which are incurred as a result of the use of the information contained within this document, including, but not limited to, errors, omissions, or inaccuracies.

Chapter 2

Acknowledgement

Thank you for your support! We truly appreciate you taking the time to read and engage with us. Your feedback means the world to us, and we'd love to hear your thoughts.

Please take a moment to scan the QR code below and share your review. Your insights help us grow and continue to provide the best experience possible.

We look forward to hearing from you, thank you again!

Chapter 3

Introduction

The Food Revolution Begins

In today's world, food is not just something we eat to survive—it's a huge part of our lives that affects our health, the environment, and even the future of our planet. How we approach food right now is more important than ever. We're at a point where the choices we make about what we eat can either make the global crisis worse or help build a healthier, more sustainable world. This is where the Food Revolution comes in—a movement aimed at changing how we eat, how we think about food, and how we treat the planet.

The Importance of Healthy, Sustainable Eating

At the heart of the Food Revolution there is an idea about how should be good for both our bodies and the environment. Eating healthy isn't just about what's good for us right now; it's about creating a lifestyle that keeps us healthy long-term, gives us energy, and helps prevent diseases. But health isn't the only thing we should think about—sustainability is equally important. The industrial food system has put a huge strain on the planet, from over-farming to the excessive use of pesticides, water waste, and high carbon emissions. When we choose food that's not only good for us but also better for the planet, we help reduce our environmental impact and make the food system more sustainable for the future.

The Impact of Food Choices on Personal Health and the Environment

The food we choose has huge consequences. On a personal level, eating nutrient-rich foods can lower our risk of chronic diseases like heart disease, diabetes, and obesity. Eating fresh fruits, vegetables, whole grains, and healthy fats gives our bodies the fuel they need to thrive. On the other hand, relying on processed and packaged foods can cause inflammation, bad gut health, and a lot of other health problems.

On a larger scale, the way we produce and consume food is a big factor in environmental damage. The demand for meat, dairy, and processed foods has caused deforestation, damaged soil, and huge water usage. If we switch to more plant-based foods, support local farmers, and buy sustainably grown food, we can cut down on our carbon footprint and fight climate change.

What to Expect from This Book

In *Food Revolution: Your Guide to Healthy, Sustainable Eating* , we'll show you how to make food choices that are good for your health and the planet. This book is here to guide you on how to embrace the Food Revolution, where you can take charge of what you eat and how you eat it. You'll learn how to build a balanced, healthy diet that fuels your body, reduce your environmental impact, and make mindful choices that support a sustainable food system.

This book will give you practical tips, easy meal-planning strategies, and simple ways to include sustainable eating habits in your daily life. From understanding the basics of nutrition to learning how to cut down on food waste, we'll cover it all. Whether you're already into healthy eating or just getting started, this book will inspire you to make thoughtful, informed decisions every time you eat.

The Food Revolution is not just a trend—it's a movement for a healthier, happier, and more sustainable life. It all starts with the choices you make at every meal. Together, we can create a food culture that supports our health, cares for the planet, and looks after future generations.

Are you ready to join the revolution? Let's get started!

Chapter 4

Understanding the Basics of Healthy Eating

Eating is one of the most essential acts of self-care we perform each day. The food we choose not only fuels our bodies but also influences our overall health, energy levels, mood, and even long-term longevity. However, in today's fast-paced world of convenience foods and quick fixes, it can be difficult to navigate through the maze of diet trends, conflicting advice, and the overwhelming number of food choices available. So, where do we begin? The answer is simple: understanding the basics of healthy eating.

The foundation of healthy eating lies in recognizing the essential nutrients our bodies require to function at their best. These nutrients can be broken down into three main categories: macro-nutrients (proteins, fats, and carbohydrates), and micro-nutrients (vitamins and minerals). This chapter will provide an in-depth exploration of each of these vital nutrients, their specific roles in the body, and how to strike a balance between them to promote health and well-being.

Essential Nutrients and Their Role in Our Body

The nutrients we consume through food play a critical role in our growth, energy production, and overall bodily functions. They can be classified into two main categories: macro-nutrients and micro-nutrients. Macro-nutrients provide energy (calories), while micronutrients help regulate various biological processes and maintain proper body function.

Macro-nutrients: Fuel for the Body

Macro-nutrients are the nutrients that our body needs in larger amounts, and they provide the energy necessary for us to live, move, and thrive. The three primary macro-nutrients are proteins, fats, and carbohydrates. While all three of these nutrients are essential for overall health, they each play different roles and should be consumed in the right proportions to maintain a balanced and healthy diet.

1. Proteins: The Building Blocks of Life

Proteins are made up of amino acids, which are the building blocks that help to build, repair, and maintain tissues in the body. They are particularly important for muscle growth and repair, immune function, enzyme production, and hormone regulation.

The Role of Protein in the Body:

- **Muscle Repair and Growth:** Proteins are crucial for the maintenance and repair of muscle tissues. This is particularly important for athletes or those who engage in regular physical activity (NIH, 2021).

- **Enzyme and Hormone Production:** Proteins are involved in the creation of enzymes, which help catalyze various biochemical reactions in the body, and hormones, which regulate bodily functions such as metabolism, mood, and stress response (Harvard T.H. Chan School of Public Health, 2022).

- **Immune System Function:** Proteins also play a critical role in immune defense, as they help form antibodies that protect the body against harmful pathogens (Mayo Clinic, 2021).

Sources of Protein:
- Animal-based sources: Chicken, turkey, beef, fish, eggs, dairy products (milk, cheese, yogurt).
- Plant-based sources: Legumes (lentils, chickpeas), beans, tofu, tempeh, quinoa, nuts, seeds, and plant-based protein powders.

How Much Protein Do You Need? The Recommended Dietary Allowance (RDA) for protein varies depending on factors like age, sex, activity level, and health goals. Generally, it's recommended that adults consume about 0.8 grams of protein per kilogram of body weight. For example, a 70 kg person would need approximately 56 grams of protein per day. For more active individuals, the requirement may be higher (National Institutes of Health, 2021).

2. Fats: Essential for Health

Contrary to common misconceptions, fats are not inherently bad. In fact, fats are essential for maintaining good health. They provide a concentrated source of energy, aid in the absorption of fat-soluble vitamins, support brain function, and promote healthy skin and hair.

The Role of Fats in the Body:
- **Energy Storage:** Fats are a concentrated source of energy. They are stored in adipose tissue and can be used when the body needs extra energy, particularly during long periods of physical activity or when carbohydrate reserves are low (American Heart Association, 2020).
- **Absorption of Vitamins:** Fat is required for the absorption of fat-soluble vitamins (A, D, E, and K), which are crucial for immune function, bone health,

and skin health (Harvard T.H. Chan School of Public Health, 2022).
- **Brain Function:** Approximately 60% of the brain is made up of fat, and consuming healthy fats supports cognitive function, memory, and mood regulation (National Institutes of Health, 2021).
- **Hormone Production:** Fat is involved in the production of hormones, including reproductive hormones, stress hormones, and metabolic regulators like insulin (American Heart Association, 2020).

Sources of Healthy Fats:
- Monounsaturated fats: Avocados, olive oil, nuts (almonds, walnuts), seeds (flaxseeds, chia seeds).
- Polyunsaturated fats: Fatty fish (salmon, mackerel), flaxseeds, walnuts, and plant oils like sunflower, safflower, and soybean oils.
- Saturated fats (in moderation): Grass-fed beef, coconut oil, dark chocolate, and dairy products.

How Much Fat Do You Need? The general recommendation is that 20-35% of your total daily calories come from fat. However, it's important to focus on the quality of fats consumed. A higher intake of unsaturated fats, and a moderate intake of saturated fats, are optimal for health (American Heart Association, 2020).

3. Carbohydrates: The Body's Primary Energy Source

Carbohydrates are the body's main source of energy. When we consume carbs, they are broken down into glucose (sugar), which the body uses as fuel for physical activity, brain function, and overall bodily processes. However, not all carbohydrates are created equal.

The Role of Carbohydrates in the Body:

- **Energy Production:** Carbs are the body's preferred source of energy, especially for the brain and muscles. When you eat carbohydrates, your body breaks them down into glucose, which circulates in the bloodstream and fuels cellular activity (Harvard T.H. Chan School of Public Health, 2022).
- **Digestive Health:** Carbohydrates, particularly fiber, play an essential role in maintaining digestive health. Fiber aids in digestion, regulates bowel movements, and supports gut microbiota (Mayo Clinic, 2021).
- **Regulation of Blood Sugar:** Carbohydrates are also essential for maintaining stable blood sugar levels. Complex carbohydrates, like whole grains, legumes, and vegetables, release glucose slowly into the bloodstream, preventing spikes and crashes in blood sugar (American Diabetes Association, 2020).

Sources of Carbohydrates:

- Complex carbohydrates: Whole grains (brown rice, oats, quinoa, barley), vegetables, legumes (lentils, beans), and fruits.
- Simple carbohydrates (preferably limited): Sugary snacks, sodas, and processed foods.

How Much Carbohydrate Do You Need? Carbohydrates should make up about 45-65% of your total daily calories. It's essential to prioritize complex carbs, which are high in fiber, over simple sugars that can lead to blood sugar imbalances (American Heart Association, 2020).

The Importance of Vitamins and Minerals

While macro-nutrients provide energy, micro-nutrients —vitamins and minerals—are essential for regulating bodily functions and preventing deficiencies. Though they are needed in smaller amounts, they are no less important.

Vitamins: Vital for Optimal Functioning

Vitamins are organic compounds that are crucial for various metabolic processes, immune function, and overall health. They are divided into two categories: fat-soluble and water-soluble.

- **Fat-soluble vitamins** (A, D, E, K) are stored in the body's fat tissues and liver. They play key roles in maintaining skin health, regulating immune function, supporting bone health, and protecting against oxidative stress (NIH, 2020).
- **Water-soluble vitamins** (C and the B vitamins) are not stored in the body and must be replenished regularly through diet. They support energy metabolism, red blood cell production, and immune function (NIH, 2020).

Minerals: The Body's Building Blocks

Minerals are inorganic substances that help with a variety of bodily functions, from building strong bones and teeth to supporting nerve function and regulating fluid balance. Key minerals include:

- **Calcium** : Supports bone health and muscle function (National Osteoporosis Foundation, 2021).
- **Iron** : Essential for transporting oxygen in the blood (National Institutes of Health, 2021).

- **Magnesium** : Involved in muscle function, nerve transmission, and energy production (National Institutes of Health, 2021).
- **Potassium** : Helps regulate fluid balance and muscle contractions (American Heart Association, 2020).

Finally, understanding the basics of healthy eating involves recognizing the importance of a balanced intake of macro-nutrients (proteins, fats, and carbohydrates) and micro-nutrients (vitamins and minerals). Each nutrient plays a unique and crucial role in supporting your body's functions, promoting optimal health, and preventing disease.

To achieve optimal health, focus on consuming a variety of whole, nutrient-dense foods that provide a mix of these essential nutrients. Aim for a balanced diet with moderate portions of protein, healthy fats, and complex carbohydrates, while ensuring you get a wide range of vitamins and minerals through colorful fruits, vegetables, and whole foods.

By mastering the basics of nutrition and making mindful choices, you can create a diet that supports both your personal well-being and the health of the planet.

Chapter 5

The Power of Whole Foods

Eating is far more than a simple necessity; it is a profound opportunity to nourish not just our bodies, but also our minds and spirits. Every bite we take impacts our overall health and well-being, influencing everything from our energy levels to our mood and even our long-term vitality. In a world where quick and convenient processed foods are often the go-to solution for busy lives, many of us have gradually moved away from the foundational principles of wholesome, nutritious eating. It's easy to fall into the trap of grabbing a fast snack or opting for a packaged meal because it's readily available. However, these choices can have long-lasting effects on our health, often leading to nutrient deficiencies, sluggish digestion, and a weakened immune system.

The good news is that we have the power to reverse these trends and take control of our health by embracing the beauty of whole foods. Whole foods—fresh, minimally processed ingredients—are packed with essential nutrients, antioxidants, and fiber, and offer a level of nourishment that processed foods simply cannot match. Whole foods provide us with the fuel we need to thrive, offering not only immediate benefits like increased energy and enhanced mental clarity but also contributing to long-term wellness by reducing the risk of chronic diseases such as heart disease, diabetes, and obesity.

In this chapter, we'll delve into the transformative power of whole foods. We will examine what whole foods truly are, why they matter for our health, and the undeniable advantages they bring to both our bodies and minds. By focusing on fresh and minimally processed foods, we'll explore how they can enhance our digestion, stabilize blood sugar levels, boost immunity, and even improve our mood and mental clarity. Additionally, we'll provide you with practical, actionable steps to help you transition smoothly to a whole-food diet—one that is sustainable and enjoyable, allowing you to reap the many benefits of nourishing your body with real, unprocessed food. Whether you're looking to improve your health, maintain a healthy weight, or simply feel better on a daily basis, embracing the power of whole foods will undoubtedly lead to lasting positive effects that will resonate throughout every aspect of your life.

What Are Whole Foods and Why Do They Matter?

At its core, whole food refers to food that is in its natural state, or close to it, without undergoing extensive processing or refinement. These foods are typically free from artificial additives, preservatives, and added sugars. In essence, whole foods are those that are minimally altered, keeping their natural nutrients intact. Whole foods can be categorized into three primary groups: fruits, vegetables, and animal products, as well as whole grains, legumes, and nuts. Let's take a closer look at some common examples of whole foods:

- **Fruits** : Apples, berries, oranges, bananas, pears
- **Vegetables** : Spinach, kale, carrots, broccoli, sweet potatoes
- **Whole Grains** : Brown rice, quinoa, oats, barley, whole-wheat bread
- **Legumes** : Beans, lentils, chickpeas, peas

- **Nuts and Seeds** : Almonds, walnuts, chia seeds, flaxseeds
- **Animal Products** : Grass-fed beef, free-range chicken, eggs, fish

Whole foods stand in contrast to processed foods, which have been altered in some way, often with the addition of refined ingredients like white flour, sugar, salt, and oils. Common processed foods include packaged snacks, frozen dinners, sugary breakfast cereals, and fast food items.

So, why do whole foods matter? The answer lies in their nutritional integrity. Whole foods retain all of their natural vitamins, minerals, fiber, and antioxidants – nutrients that are often lost during processing. For example, whole fruits are rich in fiber, which helps regulate digestion, while processed fruit juices are stripped of most of their fiber content and are often loaded with added sugar. By choosing whole foods, you are choosing to nourish your body with essential nutrients that support overall health, rather than filling up on empty calories that offer little to no nutritional value.

The Benefits of Eating Fresh, Minimally Processed Foods

The benefits of whole foods extend far beyond simply providing the nutrients your body needs. Eating fresh, minimally processed foods offers a multitude of health benefits that can significantly improve your quality of life.

- **Nutrient Density**

Whole foods are naturally nutrient-dense, meaning they provide a high concentration of vitamins, minerals, and other essential nutrients relative to their calorie content.

For example, a serving of kale provides a wealth of vitamins A, C, and K, along with fiber, calcium, and iron, all while being low in calories. In contrast, many processed foods provide empty calories with little to no nutritional value.

- **Improved Digestion**

Whole foods, particularly fruits, vegetables, whole grains, and legumes, are high in fiber, which plays an essential role in supporting a healthy digestive system. Fiber helps to regulate bowel movements, prevent constipation, and maintain a healthy gut microbiome. A diet rich in fiber can also help prevent gastrointestinal issues such as bloating and gas.

Furthermore, the gut microbiome, which consists of trillions of bacteria, is essential for overall health. A healthy, balanced microbiome is vital for digestion, immune function, and even mood regulation. Whole foods, with their natural fiber and antioxidants, promote the growth of beneficial gut bacteria, helping to keep your digestive system functioning smoothly.

- **Weight Management**

Whole foods can help with weight management by promoting satiety and reducing overeating. Unlike processed foods, which are often high in sugar and refined carbohydrates, whole foods release energy more slowly into the bloodstream, helping to stabilize blood sugar levels and curb cravings. This slow release of energy promotes feelings of fullness and reduces the likelihood of overeating, making it easier to maintain a healthy weight.

Additionally, many whole foods are lower in calories than processed foods, allowing for larger portions and more satisfying meals without overloading on calories.

For example, you can eat a large salad filled with fresh vegetables and lean protein, such as grilled chicken, without worrying about consuming excessive amounts of unhealthy fats or sugars.

- **Reduced Inflammation**

Chronic inflammation is a key contributor to many modern diseases, including heart disease, diabetes, and cancer. Processed foods, particularly those high in refined sugars, unhealthy fats, and additives, are known to promote inflammation in the body. On the other hand, whole foods, especially fruits, vegetables, and healthy fats (like those found in avocados and olive oil), contain anti-inflammatory compounds that help combat this issue.

Whole foods, such as berries, leafy greens, and fatty fish like salmon, are rich in antioxidants and omega-3 fatty acids, both of which have been shown to reduce inflammation. By incorporating these foods into your diet, you can support your body's natural ability to fight off inflammation and promote overall health.

- **Better Blood Sugar Control**

Eating whole foods that are rich in fiber and low in refined sugars helps maintain stable blood sugar levels, which is important for overall health. High blood sugar levels, especially when they occur over time, can lead to insulin resistance, type 2 diabetes, and other metabolic disorders.

Whole grains, legumes, vegetables, and fruits are low-glycemic foods, meaning they have a minimal impact on blood sugar levels. In contrast, processed foods, particularly those high in refined sugars and starches, cause rapid spikes in blood sugar, leading to crashes and cravings. By choosing whole foods, you can help keep your blood sugar levels in check and reduce your risk of developing diabetes or other chronic conditions.

- **Enhanced Mental Clarity and Mood**

Nutrition has a direct impact on brain function, mood, and mental health. Whole foods, which are rich in essential nutrients like B vitamins, antioxidants, and healthy fats, support cognitive function, reduce brain fog, and help regulate mood.

For instance, omega-3 fatty acids found in fatty fish, walnuts, and flaxseeds are essential for brain health and have been shown to help with memory, concentration, and mood regulation. Nutrients like folate and vitamin B12, found in leafy greens, legumes, and animal products, are also crucial for supporting mental clarity and emotional well-being.

By fueling your brain with whole, nutrient-dense foods, you can improve your focus, reduce feelings of anxiety and depression, and support overall cognitive health.

How to Transition to a Whole-Food Diet

Making the shift to a whole-food diet can seem daunting at first, especially if you are used to consuming a lot of processed foods. However, with a few simple steps, you can gradually transition to eating more fresh, whole foods without feeling overwhelmed.

- **Start Small**

Don't try to overhaul your entire diet overnight. Instead, start with small, manageable changes. Begin by incorporating one or two whole foods into your meals each day. For example, swap out a processed snack with a piece of fresh fruit, or replace white rice with quinoa or brown rice.

As you get used to eating whole foods, continue to increase the proportion of fresh ingredients in your meals. Over time, this will become second nature, and you'll find it easier to make healthy choices.

- **Plan Your Meals**

Meal planning is essential when transitioning to a whole-food diet. By planning your meals in advance, you can ensure that you have access to the ingredients you need, and you'll be less likely to reach for processed foods when you're hungry. Take some time each week to plan out your meals, create a grocery list, and prepare any ingredients in advance.

When meal planning, try to focus on a variety of whole foods from different food groups. Include plenty of fruits, vegetables, whole grains, legumes, nuts, and lean protein sources like chicken, fish, or tofu.

- **Cook at Home**

One of the best ways to ensure that you're eating whole foods is to cook your meals at home. When you prepare your own meals, you have full control over the ingredients, allowing you to choose fresh, unprocessed foods. Cooking at home also gives you the opportunity to experiment with new recipes and flavors, making the transition to a whole-food diet more enjoyable.

Try to cook simple, nutritious meals that are quick and easy to prepare. For example, a stir-fry made with colorful vegetables, lean protein, and brown rice is a delicious and balanced meal that can be made in under 30 minutes.

- **Read Labels**

When shopping for packaged foods, it's important to read the labels carefully. Look for items with as few ingredients as possible, and avoid those that contain artificial additives, preservatives, or added sugars. If a product has a long list of ingredients that you don't recognize, it's likely highly processed and may not be the best choice.

- **Be Patient and Persistent**

Transitioning to a whole-food diet takes time, and it's important to be patient with yourself throughout the process. Don't be discouraged if you slip up or revert back to old habits occasionally. The key is to stay persistent and continue making progress, even if it's slow. Over time, you'll begin to notice the positive effects of eating whole foods on your health and well-being.

In short, whole foods are the foundation of a healthy diet. By choosing fresh, minimally processed foods, you are providing your body with the nutrients it needs to thrive. From improved digestion and weight management to enhanced mental clarity and better blood sugar control, the benefits of eating whole foods are undeniable.

Transitioning to a whole-food diet may seem challenging at first, but with small, consistent steps, you can make the shift to a more nutritious and sustainable way of eating. By planning your meals, cooking at home, and focusing on fresh, nutrient-dense foods, you'll be well on your way to achieving optimal health and well-being.

Chapter 6

Sustainability Starts on Your Plate

In an era where environmental challenges loom large on the global stage, the urgency to adopt sustainable habits has never been greater. Among the myriad of actions we can take, the choices we make about food hold a unique and profound power. Every bite we take represents a decision that ripples across ecosystems, economies, and communities. Sustainability begins with awareness, a conscious recognition of the disconnection between our plates and the planet, and deliberate action toward protecting this fragile balance.

The concept of sustainable eating transcends mere personal health benefits—it embodies a commitment to practices that safeguard natural resources, mitigate climate change, and foster a food system that is fair, equitable, and resilient. It is about eating in a way that not only nurtures our bodies but also nurtures the Earth, reducing harm while contributing to its recovery.

This chapter embarks on an exploration of sustainable eating, highlighting its global importance in combating the ecological crises we face. It examines the far-reaching impacts of food production and consumption on our environment, including greenhouse gas emissions, water scarcity, and biodiversity loss. Moreover, it delves into critical concepts such as food miles, waste management, and resource use, offering insights into how these factors shape our environmental footprint. By understanding these dynamics, individuals are empowered to make informed decisions that align with both their values and the planet's needs.

Adopting sustainable eating practices is not just an act of responsibility but one of hope. Each mindful choice represents a step toward a future where food systems thrive in harmony with nature, communities are nourished without exploitation, and the Earth's resources are preserved for generations to come. Together, we can turn our plates into a powerful force for change.

Defining Sustainable Eating and Its Global Importance

Sustainable eating encompasses a holistic approach to consuming food that balances the needs of the present with the preservation of resources for the future. It involves choosing foods and dietary patterns that promote environmental health, economic resilience, and social equity. At its core, sustainable eating recognizes that every meal has a broader impact, extending beyond individual nourishment to influence ecosystems, communities, and economies worldwide.

This approach prioritizes practices that minimize environmental harm, such as reducing greenhouse gas emissions, conserving water, and protecting biodiversity. It also emphasizes reducing food waste and supporting ethical farming and labor practices that ensure fair treatment of workers and equitable access to nutritious food for all. Sustainable eating encourages consumers to consider the entire life cycle of their food—from production and distribution to consumption and disposal—making informed choices that align with both personal and planetary well-being.

By embracing sustainable eating, individuals contribute to creating a food system that operates within ecological boundaries, supports local economies, and upholds the dignity and rights of all involved. It's not merely a dietary preference but a commitment to fostering a harmonious relationship between humanity and the Earth, ensuring a thriving future for generations to come.

Key Principles of Sustainable Eating

1. **Local and Seasonal Foods:** Consuming food grown locally and in season reduces transportation emissions and supports local farmers.
2. **Plant-Based Focus:** Diets rich in plant-based foods and lower in animal products reduce greenhouse gas emissions and conserve water.
3. **Minimizing Waste:** From production to disposal, reducing food waste is a cornerstone of sustainability.
4. **Ethical Sourcing:** Choosing food from suppliers that follow ethical farming practices protects biodiversity and promotes fair trade.

Why It Matters Globally

The global food system is one of the largest contributors to environmental degradation. Agriculture alone accounts for 26% of global greenhouse gas emissions, with livestock production contributing nearly 15% of that total. Deforestation for agricultural expansion, excessive water use, and reliance on chemical fertilizers and pesticides further exacerbate environmental challenges. A shift toward sustainable eating habits is essential to mitigate these effects and build a resilient food system.

How Food Choices Affect the Planet

Our food choices ripple across ecosystems, economies, and communities. Understanding the environmental impact of what we eat reveals opportunities to align our habits with sustainability.

The Role of Agriculture in Climate Change

The agricultural industry is responsible for producing methane (CH_4) and nitrous oxide (N_2O), two potent greenhouse gases. Livestock farming releases methane through enteric fermentation (digestive processes in animals), while synthetic fertilizers release nitrous oxide during soil interactions. Additionally, deforestation for crops like soy and palm oil eliminates carbon sinks, further accelerating climate change.

- **Beef and Dairy:** Producing beef and dairy requires extensive land, water, and feed resources. Cows alone are responsible for nearly 10% of global greenhouse gas emissions.
- **Rice Production:** Although a staple for billions, rice paddies emit significant methane due to anaerobic decomposition in flooded fields.

Biodiversity Loss

Mono-culture farming—the practice of growing a single crop extensively—threatens biodiversity by depleting soil nutrients, increasing susceptibility to pests, and displacing native species. Deforestation to create farmland, especially in tropical regions, destroys habitats for countless species, including endangered ones.

Water Usage and Scarcity

Agriculture accounts for 70% of global freshwater withdrawals, with animal farming being particularly water-intensive. Producing one kilogram of beef requires approximately 15,400 liters of water, compared to 1,800 liters for one kilogram of wheat. In water-scarce regions, prioritizing plant-based foods and efficient irrigation techniques is crucial.

Pollution and Waste

Chemical fertilizers and pesticides pollute rivers, lakes, and groundwater, leading to algae blooms and dead zones in oceans. Additionally, packaging and food waste contribute to landfill overflow, where organic waste releases methane as it decomposes anaerobically.

Understanding Food Miles, Waste, and Resource Use

Food Miles: The Hidden Cost of Transportation

"Food miles" refer to the distance food travels from production to consumption. The longer the journey, the greater the carbon emissions associated with transportation. This metric is a critical consideration when evaluating the environmental impact of our diets.

- **Global Supply Chains:** Many imported foods require refrigeration, packaging, and extensive fuel usage during transit. For instance, tropical fruits like bananas and avocados often travel thousands of miles before reaching consumers in non-tropical regions.

- **Local Alternatives:** Opting for local, seasonal produce reduces transportation emissions and supports regional economies. For example, purchasing apples grown within 100 miles emits significantly less CO2 compared to those imported from halfway around the globe.

The Issue of Food Waste

Globally, one-third of all food produced—approximately 1.3 billion tons—is wasted annually. This waste occurs at every stage of the food supply chain, from farms and processing facilities to grocery stores and households.

- **Environmental Impact of Food Waste:** Food waste in landfills decomposes anaerobically, releasing methane—a greenhouse gas 25 times more potent than CO2.
- **Limiting Food Waste:** Solutions include smarter portioning, proper storage techniques, composting organic scraps, and donating surplus food to those in need.

Resource Use: The Energy and Water Footprint

Every step of food production requires energy and water. From growing crops and raising livestock to processing, packaging, and distribution, each stage contributes to the food's overall footprint.

- **Energy Use:** Fossil fuels are heavily relied upon for mechanized farming, refrigeration, and transportation.
- **Water Scarcity:** Regions already facing water shortages are often major exporters of water-intensive crops, further straining local resources.

Practical Steps Toward Sustainable Eating

While the challenges of building a sustainable food system are vast, individual actions collectively have a significant impact. Here are practical steps to adopt more sustainable eating habits:

Adopt a Plant-Centric Diet

Shifting the balance of your diet toward plant-based foods is one of the most effective ways to reduce your environmental impact. Incorporate more vegetables, fruits, legumes, nuts, and whole grains, and reduce reliance on meat and dairy.

Choose Local and Seasonal Produce

Seek out farmer's markets, community-supported agriculture (CSA) programs, or local grocers to find fresh, in-season produce. This reduces food miles and ensures your food is at peak freshness and nutrition.

Minimize Food Waste

Plan meals carefully, use leftovers creatively, and compost organic scraps to keep food waste out of landfills. Freezing perishable items before they spoil can also help extend their usability.

Support Sustainable Brands

Look for certifications like Fair Trade, Rain forest Alliance, and USDA Organic to identify products that align with sustainable and ethical practices. These certifications indicate environmentally friendly farming methods, fair wages, and reduced use of harmful chemicals.

Educate and Advocate

Spread awareness about sustainable eating in your community. Advocate for policies that support sustainable agriculture, food waste reduction, and the protection of natural ecosystems.

Considering all these points, sustainability truly begins on your plate. The food choices we make every day have a profound and lasting impact on the planet, shaping not only our own health but the health of the Earth itself. By understanding the principles of sustainable eating—such as choosing locally sourced, organic, and plant-based foods, supporting ethical farming practices, and minimizing food waste—we can significantly reduce our ecological footprint and contribute to a healthier, more sustainable world. Our diets are more than personal preferences; they are powerful tools that, when used intentionally, can drive meaningful change.

The effects of our food choices ripple far beyond our plates, influencing everything from greenhouse gas emissions and water use to soil health and biodiversity. Industrial agriculture, factory farming, and food production systems that prioritize profit over the planet often come at a high environmental cost. However, by adopting more sustainable eating practices, we are making a direct, positive impact. Every plant-based meal we choose, every local or organic product we support, and every piece of food we prevent from going to waste all contribute to a larger shift toward a more sustainable and resilient food system.

While systemic changes in agriculture and food production are absolutely essential for addressing the global environmental crisis, the power of individual action should not be underestimated. As consumers, we hold immense influence over the food industry. By making conscious, informed decisions about the foods we buy and consume, we can drive demand for more sustainable and ethical practices. This shift, in turn, pushes companies and farmers to adopt greener practices, reduce waste, and prioritize the planet alongside profit. Every purchase, every meal, and every habit we cultivate becomes part of a larger movement toward a food system that is healthier for both people and the planet.

Remember, every meal you eat is an opportunity to make a difference—not just for your own health, but for the future of the Earth. You have the power to contribute to a global shift toward sustainability through simple, consistent actions. Start small—whether by incorporating more plant-based meals into your diet, buying local and organic, or minimizing food waste—and gradually build these habits into your everyday life. Every positive change counts. And when you share your journey with others, you inspire collective action, helping to create a community of conscious eaters who are working together to shape a more sustainable future for all.

Your choices have the potential to influence not only your own well-being but the well-being of future generations. By embracing sustainability on your plate, you become part of a global movement toward healthier, more sustainable food systems. Start today, stay committed, and invite others to join you in making choices that benefit both our health and the planet. Together, we can create a food system that nourishes both people and the Earth, one meal at a time.

Chapter 7

The Environmental Impact of Your Diet

In today's interconnected world, the environmental consequences of human activities are alarmingly apparent, leaving profound and far-reaching impacts on our land, oceans, and atmosphere. Among the many contributors to this crisis, our dietary habits stand as one of the most significant—yet often overlooked—drivers of environmental degradation. Every stage of food production, from cultivating crops and raising livestock to processing, packaging, and distribution, exerts tremendous pressure on the planet. These activities contribute to climate change through greenhouse gas emissions, drive deforestation to make room for agricultural expansion, deplete freshwater resources through inefficient irrigation and livestock farming, and threaten global biodiversity by encroaching on natural habitats.

This unsustainable trajectory is not just a warning sign but a clear call to action. Our dietary choices hold immense power to either exacerbate or mitigate these challenges. By understanding the ecological footprint of the food we consume, we gain the insight needed to shift toward practices that nurture the planet rather than deplete it. Embracing sustainable farming techniques that replenish rather than degrade the soil, supporting ethical sourcing that prioritizes fairness and environmental care, and adopting plant-based alternatives that require fewer resources are actionable ways we can contribute to a solution.

The connection between food and the environment is more than a global issue—it is deeply personal. Every meal we eat is an opportunity to shape a more sustainable and equitable future. By making informed and intentional choices, we not only reduce our environmental impact but also inspire systemic change in the way food is grown, produced, and consumed. In our quest for nourishment, we must also nourish the Earth, ensuring its vitality for generations to come. It is through these small, collective steps that we can drive a transformative food revolution, one plate at a time.

The Carbon Footprint of Different Food Groups

A food item's carbon footprint refers to the total greenhouse gas emissions produced across its life cycle—from cultivation and processing to transportation and disposal. While all food production contributes to these emissions, the impact varies significantly between food groups.

Animal-Based Foods

Animal agriculture is responsible for approximately 14.5% of global greenhouse gas emissions, primarily through methane, carbon dioxide, and nitrous oxide. These emissions result from animal digestion, manure management, feed production, and energy-intensive practices like refrigeration and transportation.

- **Beef and Lamb:** Beef generates the highest emissions among all food items, estimated at 27 kilograms of CO_2-equivalent per kilogram produced. Lamb follows closely behind, driven by similar factors, including enteric fermentation and land use changes. For example, vast tracts of forest are cleared

to create grazing pastures, releasing stored carbon and reducing biodiversity.
- **Dairy Products:** While lower in emissions than beef, dairy products like cheese and butter are significant contributors due to methane emissions from dairy cows and the resources required to produce and process milk.
- **Poultry and Pork:** Chicken and pork production emit fewer greenhouse gases than ruminant livestock but still have a higher environmental cost than plant-based foods. Feed production, housing, and manure contribute significantly to their carbon footprint.

Plant-Based Foods

Plant-based foods generally have lower carbon footprints than animal products, although their impact can vary based on farming practices, irrigation, and transportation.

- **Grains and Pulses:** Staples such as rice, wheat, lentils, and beans are among the least carbon-intensive foods. However, rice emits methane due to anaerobic decomposition in flooded fields, making it an exception among grains.
- **Fruits and Vegetables:** These are environmentally friendly, particularly when grown locally and seasonally. Imported fruits and vegetables, or those grown in energy-intensive greenhouses, have higher emissions.
- **Nuts and Seeds:** Nuts like almonds and pistachios have a low carbon footprint but can be water-intensive. Responsible farming practices can mitigate this impact, especially in arid regions.

Processed and Packaged Foods

Highly processed foods often require significant energy for manufacturing, refrigeration, and transportation. Packaging materials, particularly single-use plastics, exacerbate the environmental burden by contributing to pollution and landfill overflow. Opting for minimally processed, bulk, or unpackaged items can help reduce waste.

Sustainable Farming and Ethical Sourcing

Sustainable agriculture and ethical sourcing aim to balance human needs with environmental health. By minimizing resource use, reducing emissions, and promoting fair labor practices, these approaches ensure long-term ecological and social well-being.

Sustainable Farming Practices

1. **Agroecology:** This farming model integrates natural ecosystems into agricultural production. Techniques such as polycultures, agroforestry, and crop rotation enhance soil fertility, reduce pests, and support biodiversity.

2. **Water Management:** With agriculture consuming 70% of global freshwater resources, sustainable practices like drip irrigation, rainwater harvesting, and mulching are essential for conserving water.

3. **Carbon Sequestration:** Certain practices, such as no-till farming, cover cropping, and reforestation, actively capture and store carbon in soil and vegetation, mitigating climate change.

4. **Regenerative Agriculture:** Beyond sustainability, regenerative farming focuses on restoring degraded

soils, increasing biodiversity, and enhancing water cycles. This approach is gaining traction among progressive farms worldwide.

Ethical Sourcing

Ethical sourcing ensures that food production respects the environment, workers, and animals. Key certifications and practices include:

- **Fair Trade:** Ensures fair wages, safe working conditions, and community development in farming regions, particularly in developing countries.
- **Animal Welfare Standards:** Certifications like Certified Humane and Animal Welfare Approved promote humane treatment of animals, including access to pasture and elimination of overcrowding.
- **Locally Sourced Foods:** Supporting local farms reduces transportation emissions, strengthens local economies, and provides fresher, seasonal produce.

How Plant-Based Diets Contribute to Sustainability

Transitioning to a plant-based diet is one of the most effective ways to reduce the environmental footprint of food production. By relying on foods that require fewer resources and produce fewer emissions, individuals can make a significant impact.

Greenhouse Gas Reduction

Animal agriculture is responsible for the majority of emissions in the food sector, including methane from livestock and nitrous oxide from fertilizers. Switching to plant-based proteins like lentils, tofu, and beans can cut emissions dramatically. Studies suggest that adopting a plant-based diet globally could reduce greenhouse gas emissions by up to 70%.

Efficient Land Use

Producing plant-based foods requires less land than raising livestock. For example, soybeans grown for direct human consumption use a fraction of the land required to produce beef or pork. Freeing up land previously used for animal agriculture allows for rewilding and carbon sequestration through reforestation.

Water Conservation

Meat and dairy production are among the most water-intensive food systems. By comparison, most plant-based foods require significantly less water. For instance, producing one pound of beef consumes approximately 1,800 gallons of water, whereas the same amount of tofu requires only about 300 gallons.

Preserving Biodiversity

Deforestation for cattle ranching and feed production is a leading driver of habitat destruction and biodiversity loss. By reducing demand for meat, we can slow deforestation and protect endangered species. Plant-based diets also reduce the need for monoculture crops like corn and soy, which can deplete soil and harm local ecosystems.

Making Sustainable Food Choices

Adopting sustainable eating habits doesn't require a complete dietary overhaul overnight. Small, incremental changes can lead to substantial benefits for the environment:

1. **Start Small:** Try implementing "Meatless Mondays" or adding one plant-based meal per day.
2. **Prioritize Local and Seasonal Foods:** Local produce requires less transportation and supports regional farmers. Seasonal foods reduce the need for energy-intensive storage and hothouses.
3. **Minimize Waste:** Plan meals carefully, use leftovers creatively, and compost organic waste to reduce landfill emissions.
4. **Opt for Sustainable Brands:** Look for certifications like USDA Organic, Rain forest Alliance, and Fair Trade on packaged products.
5. **Educate and Advocate:** Share your knowledge about sustainable eating with friends and family to inspire broader change.

In the end, the environmental impact of our diets is one of the most powerful yet often overlooked aspects of climate action. Our food choices—what we eat, where it comes from, and how it is produced—play a significant role in shaping the health of our planet. By understanding the carbon footprint of various food groups, supporting sustainable farming practices, prioritizing ethical sourcing, and incorporating more plant-based options into our meals, we can significantly reduce our ecological impact and contribute to the health of the planet.

The production of food is responsible for a large proportion of greenhouse gas emissions, deforestation, water depletion, and soil degradation. By making informed and conscious food choices, we can decrease these harmful environmental effects. For instance, plant-based foods generally have a much lower carbon footprint than animal-based foods, as they require fewer resources to produce and cause less pollution. Incorporating more plant-based meals into our diets is one of the simplest and most effective ways to reduce our carbon footprint and help mitigate climate change.

Supporting sustainable farming methods and ethical sourcing practices is another powerful tool in building a more sustainable food system. Sustainable farming prioritizes the health of the soil, the preservation of biodiversity, and the conservation of natural resources, all of which help reduce environmental degradation. Ethical sourcing ensures that food is produced under fair labor practices, minimizing exploitation and ensuring equitable access for all. By choosing to support local farmers, organic growers, and fair-trade producers, we help promote a system that values the environment, the people who cultivate the land, and the long-term health of our ecosystems.

The choices we make today—whether in the foods we eat, the brands we support, or the farming methods we choose to prioritize—shape the future of our environment. Every small action, from reducing food waste to choosing sustainable and plant-based options, adds up to create meaningful change. When we consider the environmental cost of the food we consume and take steps to make more mindful, eco-friendly choices, we actively contribute to the creation of a sustainable world. The impact of these individual decisions can help protect the planet, safeguard resources for future generations, and ensure a healthier, more vibrant ecosystem for years to come. In the quest for a sustainable future, every meal, every choice, and every effort counts.

Chapter 8

Decoding Labels: What You Need to Know

In today's food marketplace, where grocery shelves are overflowing with a dizzying variety of products, making informed and healthy choices can feel like an overwhelming challenge. Every aisle presents a vast array of options—each boasting a unique combination of nutritional claims, ingredient lists, and certifications. Labels on food packaging are supposed to simplify our purchasing decisions, but they often seem like a maze of information designed to cater to every trend, health fad, and marketing strategy. From "low-fat" to "sugar-free" and from "superfoods" to "all-natural," it's easy to become confused or misled.

For many consumers, understanding these labels requires more than just basic knowledge; it demands a deeper understanding of what's truly in our food and the broader impact these choices have on our bodies and the planet. Behind the alluring claims and flashy logos, there's often more than meets the eye. This chapter is dedicated to demystifying the art of decoding food labels. It provides the essential tools to not only read nutrition facts and ingredient lists, but also to critically analyze certifications like Organic, Fair Trade, and Non-GMO, and understand what these really mean for both your health and the environment.

We'll explore how to identify red flags and hidden sugars, the significance of portion sizes, and why certain ingredients make the cut in some products while others don't. Additionally, we'll examine the environmental, ethical, and social dimensions of your food choices by diving into labels that indicate sustainable practices and ethical sourcing. Armed with this knowledge, you'll be empowered to make more conscious decisions, selecting foods that not only nourish your body but also contribute to a healthier, more sustainable, and fairer food system. By the end of this chapter, you'll have the tools and confidence to navigate today's complex food labels with clarity and purpose, ensuring that your shopping cart reflects both your health goals and values.

How to Read Nutrition Labels and Ingredient Lists

Food labels provide a snapshot of what's inside a product, helping consumers evaluate its nutritional content and quality. However, navigating these labels requires some understanding of their structure and terminology.

The Nutrition Facts Panel

The nutrition facts panel is standardized in most countries and provides critical information about the nutrient content of a food product. Here's a breakdown of its key components:

1. **Serving Size:**
    - The serving size is the foundation for understanding the rest of the nutrition information. All data on the label—calories, fats, protein, vitamins, and minerals—are based on this portion.
    - Be mindful that the serving size might not reflect the amount you typically consume. For instance, a bag of chips might list nutritional data for a single serving, but the bag contains multiple servings.

3. **Calories:**
   - This figure represents the energy provided by one serving. While calorie needs vary depending on age, gender, and activity level, excessive calorie consumption can lead to weight gain.
5. **Macronutrients:**
   - **Fats:** The label distinguishes between saturated fats, trans fats, and unsaturated fats. While unsaturated fats are heart-healthy, saturated and trans fats should be limited to reduce the risk of heart disease.
   - **Carbohydrates:** This includes sugars, fiber, and starches. High dietary fiber is beneficial for digestion, while added sugars should be minimized.
   - **Protein:** Protein content is crucial for muscle repair and overall health, especially for active individuals.
7. **Micronutrients:**
   - These include vitamins and minerals like calcium, iron, vitamin D, and potassium. Adequate intake supports various body functions and helps prevent deficiencies.
9. **% Daily Value (%DV):**
   - This percentage indicates how much a nutrient in one serving contributes to the average daily requirement based on a 2,000-calorie diet. Values of 5% or less are considered low, while 20% or more is high.

Ingredient Lists

The ingredient list is a critical element of any food label, offering a detailed breakdown of the product's components in descending order by weight. This list serves as an essential tool for consumers, providing valuable insight into the quality and composition of a food product. By carefully examining the ingredient list, you can identify not only the primary ingredients but also potentially harmful additives, artificial substances, allergens, and preservatives that might be lurking in the product.

The order of ingredients matters—items listed at the top of the list represent the largest proportion of the product, while those near the end are present in smaller quantities. This hierarchy allows you to quickly assess the overall quality of a product. For example, if sugar, high-fructose corn syrup, or refined oils appear near the top of the list, it signals that the product is likely highly processed and less nutritious. On the other hand, a product that starts with whole grains, fresh fruits, or natural proteins suggests a healthier, more wholesome option.

The ingredient list also serves as a key tool for identifying allergens such as peanuts, gluten, dairy, or soy, which are often highlighted by food manufacturers due to their potential health risks. Understanding these components allows you to make more informed choices, particularly if you are managing food sensitivities, allergies, or specific dietary preferences. Ultimately, the ingredient list is your roadmap to discerning the true value of the product, helping you avoid unnecessary additives while selecting foods that are more aligned with your health and sustainability goals.

1. **Spotting Added Sugars:**
   - Added sugars can appear under many names, including sucrose, high-fructose corn syrup, and agave nectar. Limiting these is key to avoiding empty calories.
3. **Avoiding Harmful Additives:**
   - Artificial preservatives, colorings, and flavorings may pose health risks or indicate a highly processed product. Watch for terms like sodium benzoate, monosodium glutamate (MSG), and artificial dyes.
5. **Understanding Buzzwords:**
   - Labels like "natural" and "multigrain" can be misleading, as they are not strictly regulated. Reading the full ingredient list provides a clearer picture of a product's quality.

Understanding Certifications: Organic, Fair Trade, and Non-GMO

Certifications are another critical aspect of food labels, offering insight into how a product was produced. These labels reflect environmental, social, and ethical considerations, helping consumers align purchases with their values.

Organic Certification

Organic products are grown and processed according to strict regulations designed to promote ecological balance and avoid synthetic inputs. Key aspects include:

- **No Synthetic Pesticides or Fertilizers:** Organic farming prioritizes natural methods for pest control and soil enrichment.
- **No Genetically Modified Organisms (GMOs):** Organic certification prohibits the use of GMOs in crops or animal feed.
- **Animal Welfare Standards:** Organic livestock must be raised in humane conditions, with access to pasture and organic feed.

Pros of Organic Products:

- Lower pesticide residues compared to conventionally grown produce.
- Better for soil health and biodiversity.
- Free from synthetic hormones and antibiotics in the case of animal products.

Limitations of Organic Certification:

- Organic doesn't always mean healthier; some organic products are high in sugar, fat, or salt.
- Organic farming requires more land and can have a higher carbon footprint per unit of food in certain cases.

Fair Trade Certification

Fair Trade focuses on ethical sourcing, ensuring that farmers and workers receive fair wages and work in safe conditions. Key benefits include:

- **Economic Support for Farmers:** Fair Trade premiums are invested in community development and sustainable farming initiatives.
- **Environmental Practices:** Many Fair Trade-certified farms also employ sustainable techniques to reduce their environmental impact.
- **Product Scope:** Fair Trade certification is common in commodities like coffee, chocolate, bananas, and tea.

What to Watch For:
Not all Fair Trade-certified products are organic, so it's important to check for both labels if sustainability is a concern.

Non-GMO Certification

The Non-GMO Project certification assures consumers that a product is free from genetically modified organisms. While GMOs are safe to eat, concerns about their environmental impact, such as increased pesticide use, drive demand for Non-GMO products.

Key Features:

- Verified Non-GMO products avoid genetic engineering in crops and animal feed.
- Common Non-GMO crops include corn, soy, and canola.

Considerations:
- Non-GMO certification does not guarantee organic or sustainable farming practices.

Choosing Products with Minimal Environmental Impact

Food production stands as one of the most significant contributors to environmental degradation, with far-reaching consequences for our planet. From greenhouse gas emissions and water scarcity to deforestation and habitat destruction, the way we grow, process, and consume food has a profound effect on the health of our ecosystems. The agricultural industry is responsible for a substantial portion of global carbon emissions, much of which comes from practices like livestock farming, monocropping, and the overuse of synthetic fertilizers and pesticides. Additionally, the massive demand for water in food production exacerbates the growing problem of water scarcity, while industrial farming and food processing contribute to soil erosion, water pollution, and biodiversity loss.

In light of these challenges, making food choices that minimize environmental impact becomes crucial. It requires a more holistic approach that goes beyond just the ingredients on the label, incorporating considerations such as the sourcing, packaging, and processing methods of the products we purchase. By opting for sustainable farming practices, reducing packaging waste, and supporting responsible sourcing, consumers can help drive positive environmental change and reduce their ecological footprint.

Sourcing is one of the most impactful ways to ensure your food choices have minimal environmental impact. Locally sourced products generally require fewer resources to transport, reducing emissions tied to food miles. Furthermore, supporting sustainable farming practices that prioritize soil health, biodiversity, and water conservation can help mitigate environmental damage. In addition, products that are certified organic, Fair Trade, or Non-GMO often come from farms that employ environmentally friendly methods, such as crop rotation, agroforestry, and reduced chemical use, helping to preserve ecosystems and reduce pollution.

Packaging also plays a critical role in determining the environmental impact of a food product. Excessive plastic packaging, single-use containers, and non-recyclable materials contribute to growing landfills and oceans filled with plastic waste. Choosing products with minimal or eco-friendly packaging, such as biodegradable or recyclable materials, significantly reduces waste and supports a circular economy. In addition, buying in bulk and choosing loose produce instead of pre-packaged options can drastically cut down on packaging waste.

Lastly, **processing** —the methods used to prepare and manufacture food—can also influence its environmental impact. Highly processed foods often require more energy, water, and chemicals during production, contributing to pollution and resource depletion. On the other hand, minimally processed foods, such as fresh fruits and vegetables, whole grains, and unrefined plant-based products, tend to have a lower environmental footprint. Opting for foods that require less industrial processing not only supports your health but also reduces the strain on the planet's resources.

Ultimately, the way we choose our food is a powerful tool for reducing environmental degradation. By considering the full life cycle of the products we consume—how they are grown, processed, packaged, and transported—we can make more sustainable choices that align with our health goals and contribute to a healthier planet. Every conscious decision, from buying local to choosing responsibly sourced ingredients, plays a part in building a food system that values the Earth and all its inhabitants.

Packaging and Waste

- **Minimal Packaging:** Opt for products with little to no packaging, or packaging made from recyclable or biodegradable materials.
- **Bulk Buying:** Purchasing items in bulk reduces the amount of packaging waste.

Local and Seasonal Foods

- **Reducing Food Miles:** Locally sourced products reduce emissions from transportation. Look for "locally grown" labels or shop at farmers' markets.
- **Seasonality:** Seasonal produce requires fewer artificial growing conditions and supports regional agriculture.

Support Brands with Environmental Commitments

- Look for brands with certifications like Certified B Corporation, which measures social and environmental performance.
- Research companies that prioritize sustainability through renewable energy, reduced emissions, and transparent supply chains.

Focus on Plant-Based Foods

Plant-based diets generally have a lower environmental footprint than diets centered on animal products. Choosing products like legumes, grains, and locally grown fruits and vegetables supports sustainable eating.

As a result, decoding food labels is an essential skill for making informed, ethical, and environmentally conscious choices. By understanding the nutrition facts panel, ingredient lists, and certifications, consumers can navigate the complex food landscape with confidence. Moreover, prioritizing products with minimal environmental impact ensures that our choices benefit not only our health but also the planet. Every item placed in a shopping cart represents a vote for the kind of world we want to live in—a world where health, sustainability, and fairness guide our decisions.

Chapter 9

Building a Sustainable Pantry

A well-stocked pantry does more than just provide the necessary ingredients for cooking—it forms the very foundation of a healthy and sustainable lifestyle. In a world increasingly aware of the environmental and health challenges we face, the foods we choose to keep in our kitchen can have a far-reaching impact. By filling our pantries with eco-friendly, organic, and locally-sourced staples, we are not only making thoughtful choices about the meals we prepare, but we are also reducing our environmental footprint, supporting ethical farming practices, and contributing to a more sustainable food system. Every ingredient in your pantry is an opportunity to make a positive change—whether it's for your health, the planet, or the future of sustainable eating.

In today's world, food choices extend beyond just taste or convenience; they are deeply intertwined with the planet's well-being. The way food is produced, transported, and consumed has a direct effect on the environment—affecting everything from carbon emissions and water use to deforestation, biodiversity loss, and pollution. By focusing on sustainable, health-conscious ingredients, we are not only fueling our bodies with nutrient-dense foods but also making an impact on the systems that govern how food reaches our tables. A sustainable pantry, then, becomes much more than a simple collection of foods—it is a reflection of a conscious commitment to environmental and personal well-being.

This chapter is designed to help you build a sustainable pantry, one that supports both your health and the planet. We will explore the key principles of creating an eco-conscious pantry, starting with the fundamental elements of selecting healthy, nutrient-rich foods. From whole grains and legumes to plant-based proteins and seasonal produce, we'll look at the pantry staples that should form the backbone of your kitchen. In addition, we'll delve into sourcing organic and local ingredients, exploring how these choices support ethical farming practices and reduce the negative environmental impact of industrial agriculture. Along with these ingredient-focused strategies, we will also examine the importance of reducing food waste by shopping mindfully, buying in bulk, and learning proper food storage techniques to extend the life of your pantry items.

Stocking Your Kitchen with Healthy, Eco-Friendly Staples

The first step to building a sustainable pantry is understanding the types of ingredients that are both healthy for you and less harmful to the environment. These ingredients should ideally be nutrient-dense, minimally processed, and produced in ways that conserve resources and minimize pollution. Let's explore the key categories of eco-friendly staples to stock up on, focusing on their nutritional benefits and environmental impact.

Whole Grains

Whole grains are the foundation of a healthy, sustainable pantry. They are rich in fiber, vitamins, and minerals, and their cultivation generally has a lower environmental impact than refined grains. Whole grains such as brown rice, quinoa, farro, oats, and barley are nutrient-packed options that can form the base of numerous dishes.

- **Environmental Benefits:** Growing whole grains typically requires fewer inputs in terms of pesticides, fertilizers, and irrigation compared to animal products. Moreover, many whole grains, such as oats and barley, are drought-tolerant and grow well in diverse climates, making them resilient to changing weather patterns.
- **Health Benefits:** Whole grains are known for improving digestive health, stabilizing blood sugar levels, and reducing the risk of chronic diseases like heart disease and diabetes.

Tip: Opt for whole grains in bulk to reduce packaging waste and save money.

Legumes and Pulses

Beans, lentils, chickpeas, and peas are some of the most eco-friendly, protein-packed staples you can keep in your pantry. These plant-based proteins are affordable, versatile, and provide significant health benefits.

- **Environmental Benefits:** Legumes and pulses have a low carbon footprint compared to animal-based proteins. They require little water and can fix nitrogen in the soil, which improves soil health and reduces the need for synthetic fertilizers. Furthermore, they typically have fewer greenhouse gas emissions during cultivation.
- **Health Benefits:** Rich in protein, fiber, and various micronutrients like iron and folate, legumes are essential for heart health, weight management, and maintaining healthy blood sugar levels.

Tip: Choose dry beans or pulses over canned versions to reduce packaging waste and cost.

Nuts and Seeds

Nuts like almonds, walnuts, and cashews, as well as seeds such as chia, flax, and sunflower, are packed with healthy fats, protein, and essential vitamins. When stored properly, they have a long shelf life, making them perfect for pantry stocking.

- **Environmental Benefits:** Nuts and seeds have a relatively low environmental impact compared to animal-derived protein sources. While nuts such as almonds require water-intensive farming, their carbon footprint is still much lower than meat production. Additionally, they require far fewer resources compared to animal-based protein sources.
- **Health Benefits:** Rich in heart-healthy omega-3 fatty acids, protein, and fiber, nuts and seeds are excellent for promoting cardiovascular health, supporting brain function, and providing energy.

Tip: Buy in bulk and store nuts and seeds in airtight containers to preserve freshness and minimize waste.

Canned and Frozen Vegetables and Fruits

When fresh produce is not available, canned and frozen vegetables and fruits are excellent alternatives. They retain much of their nutritional value and provide convenience without compromising your sustainable living goals.

- **Environmental Benefits:** Canned and frozen fruits and vegetables often have a lower carbon footprint than fresh produce, especially if you buy them in bulk or choose products grown locally.

Freezing or canning produce reduces spoilage, extending the life of food and reducing waste.

- **Health Benefits:** Frozen and canned vegetables and fruits are a great way to increase your intake of vitamins, minerals, and fiber, particularly when fresh produce is out of season.

Tip: Opt for varieties with no added sugar, salt, or preservatives to ensure that you're getting the healthiest option possible.

Organic and Local Options for Long-Term Pantry Essentials

One of the most powerful ways to reduce the environmental impact of your pantry is by prioritizing organic and locally sourced products. Organic farming methods avoid the use of harmful synthetic pesticides and fertilizers, which can damage ecosystems, pollute water supplies, and contribute to soil degradation. By opting for organic, you are supporting farming practices that focus on building healthy, fertile soil, enhancing biodiversity, and promoting the long-term sustainability of our natural resources. Organic farms tend to emphasize crop rotation, natural pest management, and reduced reliance on non-renewable resources, which helps maintain ecological balance and protect the environment.

In addition, sourcing food locally is an impactful way to further reduce your ecological footprint. When food is grown and produced locally, it doesn't require the extensive transportation typically involved in importing goods from distant regions or countries. This reduction in transportation leads to fewer greenhouse gas emissions, lower fuel consumption, and reduced packaging waste. Local produce also tends to be harvested at its peak ripeness, which means it's fresher, more nutrient-dense, and often tastier than foods that have traveled long distances. By supporting local farmers and food producers, you also contribute to the vitality of local economies and help build more resilient food systems.

Choosing organic and locally grown foods is not just about personal health—it's a collective commitment to nurturing the planet. With every meal, you can make a positive environmental impact, helping to protect the soil, air, and water resources that sustain life. Moreover, by reducing the carbon emissions associated with transportation and supporting more sustainable growing practices, you're taking meaningful steps toward creating a more sustainable food system for future generations.

Why Organic?

Organic foods are grown without the use of synthetic chemicals, antibiotics, or genetically modified organisms (GMOs). Organic farming practices are designed to support soil health, conserve water, reduce pollution, and protect biodiversity. By choosing organic pantry staples, you're supporting farming systems that prioritize ecological health and sustainability.

- **Environmental Benefits:** Organic farming practices encourage crop diversity, reduce pesticide use, and often involve techniques that improve soil structure and increase water retention.
- **Health Benefits:** Organic foods are free from harmful chemicals, which may reduce exposure to pesticides and additives. They also tend to have higher levels of antioxidants and essential nutrients.

Tip: Focus on the Environmental Working Group's (EWG) "Dirty Dozen" and "Clean Fifteen" lists when choosing organic produce to prioritize which items are worth purchasing organically.

Supporting Local Producers

Buying local has significant environmental and social benefits. When you buy locally produced foods, you reduce the carbon emissions associated with food transportation and support your local economy.

- **Environmental Benefits:** Local foods require less packaging and less transportation, both of which reduce the carbon footprint of your food. Moreover, many local farms use more sustainable practices, such as crop rotation, reduced pesticide use, and smaller-scale production.

- **Health Benefits:** Local produce is often fresher and has a higher nutrient content, as it spends less time in transit. By purchasing directly from local farmers, you can ensure that your food is grown without harmful chemicals and pesticides.

Tip: Shop at farmers' markets, join a community-supported agriculture (CSA) program, or visit local co-ops to find fresh, locally-grown pantry staples.

How to Reduce Food Waste Through Mindful Buying

One of the most impactful ways to make your pantry more sustainable is by reducing food waste. Each year, millions of tons of food are discarded due to overbuying, improper storage, and inefficient meal planning. By being mindful of how we purchase and store food, we can significantly cut down on waste and reduce the demand for additional agricultural resources.

Plan Your Meals

One of the most effective ways to reduce food waste is by planning your meals in advance. By creating a shopping list based on your meals for the week, you can avoid impulse buys and unnecessary food items that may go to waste.

- **Environmental Benefits:** By reducing waste, you minimize the need for additional food production, transportation, and disposal. Less food waste means fewer resources are spent on growing, packaging, and transporting items that ultimately never get consumed.
- **Health Benefits:** Meal planning helps you create balanced meals, ensuring you get the proper nutrients. It also allows you to rotate pantry items, reducing the likelihood of them expiring before use.

Tip: Batch cook meals and freeze leftovers to reduce the temptation of ordering take-out or purchasing more ingredients than needed.

Buy in Bulk

Buying pantry staples in bulk helps minimize packaging waste and can save you money. Bulk buying allows you to purchase only the quantities you need, which can also reduce food spoilage and waste.

- **Environmental Benefits:** Bulk purchasing eliminates the need for excessive packaging and plastic, which contributes to landfill waste and pollution.

- **Health Benefits:** By buying in bulk, you can select the freshest, most nutrient-rich ingredients, and you can tailor your purchases to avoid food spoilage.

Tip: Invest in reusable bags or containers to store bulk items such as grains, legumes, and dried fruits, reducing your reliance on single-use packaging.

Proper Storage and Preservation

Properly storing your pantry items is key to minimizing food waste. Many foods, such as grains, nuts, and legumes, can be kept for long periods, but they must be stored in airtight containers to prevent spoilage and pests.

- **Environmental Benefits:** Proper storage extends the life of your pantry items, reducing the frequency of food waste and the need for constant replenishment.
- **Health Benefits:** Proper storage keeps your pantry items fresh and safe to eat, ensuring that you're not consuming expired or spoiled food.

Tip: Label your pantry items with the purchase date to keep track of their shelf life and rotate older items to the front to use them before they expire.

Finally, building a sustainable pantry is not just a practical aspect of daily life—it's a powerful step toward living a more eco-conscious and health-focused lifestyle. When you stock your pantry with eco-friendly, organic, and locally sourced ingredients, you are actively making food choices that reflect your commitment to the environment and the planet's well-being. These ingredients, often cultivated with minimal use of harmful pesticides and fertilizers, promote healthier soil, cleaner water, and reduced environmental degradation. Organic farming methods emphasize sustainability, biodiversity, and soil health—ensuring that the food you consume supports the long-term balance of our ecosystems.

Furthermore, when you choose to purchase locally grown foods, you reduce the carbon footprint associated with long-distance food transportation. Local food systems typically require less energy, fewer resources, and lower emissions, making them an essential part of building a sustainable and resilient food supply. Locally sourced ingredients also tend to be fresher, more nutrient-dense, and often more flavorful, making them a healthier choice for your body and your taste buds.

Beyond sourcing the right foods, adopting mindful practices that minimize food waste is equally important in creating a truly sustainable pantry. By integrating strategies like meal planning, buying in bulk, and proper food storage, you can ensure that the ingredients you bring into your home are used efficiently, reducing unnecessary waste and excess. Meal planning helps you purchase only what you need, reducing the likelihood of forgotten ingredients going unused and being discarded. Buying in bulk reduces packaging waste and allows you to purchase just the right amount, minimizing food spoilage and waste. Proper storage techniques, such as vacuum sealing or using airtight containers, extend the shelf life of your pantry staples, ensuring that nothing goes to waste.

The heart of a sustainable pantry lies in making intentional and mindful purchasing decisions. It's about more than just buying organic or local; it's about choosing food that supports both personal health and environmental integrity. By being deliberate in your food choices and actively reducing waste, you are contributing to a system of consumption that values the health of both the planet and yourself. Every conscious decision, from selecting eco-friendly ingredients to reducing food waste, has a ripple effect that supports sustainable food systems, healthier ecosystems, and a more vibrant future for generations to come. A sustainable pantry is a tangible way to take action—one meal at a time—for a healthier planet and a healthier you.

Chapter 10

Meal Planning for Health and Sustainability

Meal planning is not just a practical approach to organizing our meals—it's an essential practice with far-reaching benefits that can significantly improve our personal health and contribute to the well-being of the planet. In today's fast-paced, convenience-driven world, meal planning and prepping may seem like an additional burden or time-consuming task. However, when we understand the myriad advantages of planning ahead—from improved nutrition and reduced food waste to cost savings and a lower environmental impact—it becomes evident that investing a little time in meal preparation can yield profound rewards. Thoughtful meal planning enables us to make healthier, more mindful choices, helping us take control of what we eat while also supporting a sustainable food system.

By taking the time to plan our meals, we empower ourselves to make better choices, not just for our bodies, but for the planet as well. Whether it's choosing local, seasonal produce or reducing food waste, every small decision can lead to a more sustainable and resilient food system. Through deliberate meal planning, we can reduce our reliance on convenience foods that are often nutritionally poor and environmentally taxing, and instead embrace healthier, nutrient-rich meals that are both satisfying and sustainable. In this way, meal planning becomes an act of both self-care and environmental stewardship.

This chapter will delve into the key elements of successful meal planning: from the importance of meal prepping ahead of time to the steps for creating balanced, nutritious meals that support our health and well-being. Additionally, we will explore how sustainable meal planning practices can help reduce food waste, save money, and minimize our ecological footprint. Throughout, we will provide practical, actionable strategies and tips to make meal planning easier, more effective, and more beneficial to both you and the planet. Whether you're new to meal planning or looking to refine your approach, this chapter will equip you with the tools you need to transform your eating habits into something that promotes long-term health and sustainability.

The Importance of Meal Prepping and Planning Ahead

Meal planning is an intentional strategy that offers a wide range of benefits, from better physical health to more sustainable consumption patterns. When we meal plan, we take the guesswork out of our daily food choices, which results in healthier, more mindful eating.

Health Benefits of Meal Planning

One of the primary benefits of meal planning is that it provides the opportunity to make conscious, healthy food choices. Without a plan, we may rely on convenience foods, takeout, or unhealthy processed options that can contribute to excess calories, sugar, unhealthy fats, and sodium. Meal planning allows us to prioritize whole, nutrient-dense foods—such as fresh fruits and vegetables, whole grains, lean proteins, and healthy fats—ensuring we meet our nutritional needs.

Having meals planned ahead of time ensures that every dish is balanced, with the proper portions of macronutrients—proteins, fats, and carbohydrates—

while also meeting micronutrient needs. The benefit of meal prepping is that it removes the temptation to skip meals or reach for processed snacks, helping to maintain consistent, balanced nutrition throughout the day. For instance, a well-planned lunch of grilled chicken with quinoa and steamed vegetables provides lean protein, fiber-rich grains, and essential vitamins and minerals— all necessary for maintaining energy, supporting immunity, and managing blood sugar levels.

Moreover, meal planning supports portion control. By preparing meals ahead of time, we can eliminate the guesswork around portion sizes, reducing overeating or under-eating. When meals are pre-portioned, we are better able to keep our calorie intake in check, which is vital for those focused on weight management or improving specific health conditions like diabetes or heart disease.

Reducing Stress and Improving Time Management

In addition to promoting healthy eating, meal planning reduces daily stress around food choices. Many people face decision fatigue after a long workday or hectic schedule, and the last thing they want to do is figure out what to eat. Planning meals ahead of time eliminates this pressure, allowing us to focus on other priorities. By taking just a small amount of time each week to plan meals, we free ourselves from the stress of last-minute decisions or resorting to takeout or convenience foods, which often come with a higher cost and a lower nutritional value.

Meal prepping also helps save time during the week. Preparing multiple meals in one session means we don't need to spend time cooking every single day. With pre-made lunches and dinners, we can simply heat and serve, saving us valuable time. For families, this can be particularly helpful when juggling busy schedules, as the time spent cooking can be reduced, and the risk of unhealthy or rushed meal choices diminishes.

Financial Savings

While it may seem that meal planning requires extra effort, in reality, it saves both time and money. By planning meals ahead of time, we reduce impulse buys, which are often made in the grocery store or when faced with hunger and lack of meal options. The strategic planning of meals allows us to make efficient shopping lists, avoid waste, and take advantage of bulk purchases. For example, buying grains and legumes in bulk can reduce overall food costs.

Another important aspect is reducing food waste. One of the major causes of wasted money in the kitchen is buying food we don't end up using. Meal planning ensures we purchase only what we need for the week, minimizing the likelihood of unused, expired food items in the fridge. According to the Food and Agriculture Organization (FAO), nearly a third of the food produced worldwide is wasted, and a significant portion of that waste occurs in homes. By reducing food waste through better planning, we can save money while also contributing to a more sustainable food system.

How to Create Balanced, Nutritious Meals

Creating balanced meals is at the core of meal planning. A well-rounded meal provides all the essential nutrients the body needs, including proteins, healthy fats, carbohydrates, vitamins, and minerals. A balanced plate helps maintain energy levels, supports brain function, and promotes overall wellness. Below, we'll outline some key strategies for building balanced, nutritious meals.

Understanding Macronutrients

Macronutrients—proteins, fats, and carbohydrates—are the primary nutrients our bodies need in large amounts to function properly. Understanding the role of each macronutrient is crucial to designing meals that fuel the body effectively.

1. **Proteins:** Proteins are necessary for building and repairing tissues, making enzymes, and supporting immune function. A balanced meal should include a source of lean protein such as chicken, fish, tofu, beans, lentils, or eggs. Plant-based proteins, in particular, are a great choice for supporting sustainability, as they generally have a lower environmental footprint compared to animal-based proteins.

2. **Healthy Fats:** Healthy fats play an important role in the body's cell structure, energy storage, and absorption of fat-soluble vitamins. Including a source of healthy fats—such as avocado, olive oil, nuts, or seeds—provides long-lasting energy and supports heart health.

3. **Carbohydrates:** Carbs are the body's primary energy source. Choose complex carbohydrates like whole grains (quinoa, brown rice, oats), starchy vegetables (sweet potatoes, butternut squash), and legumes (lentils, chickpeas). These foods provide fiber, which is essential for digestive health and helps maintain stable blood sugar levels.

Micronutrients and the Importance of Variety

Micronutrients—vitamins and minerals—are just as essential for health as macronutrients, even though they are needed in smaller amounts. To ensure a balanced meal plan, it is important to include a wide variety of vegetables, fruits, and other nutrient-dense foods. Different colors in fruits and vegetables often indicate a variety of nutrients, so aim for a rainbow on your plate.

- **Leafy greens** like spinach, kale, and Swiss chard are excellent sources of iron, calcium, and magnesium.
- **Citrus fruits** such as oranges, lemons, and grapefruits are packed with vitamin C, which supports immune function.
- **Berries** provide antioxidants that help protect cells from damage and reduce inflammation.
- **Root vegetables** like carrots, beets, and sweet potatoes are rich in vitamins A and C, and they also provide important fiber.

Building Your Meal: A Simple Guide

When it comes to meal building, a simple method is to follow the "half-plate" rule, ensuring that half your plate is filled with vegetables and fruits, a quarter with protein, and the other quarter with healthy grains or carbohydrates. This ensures that you're getting a nutrient-dense meal that offers a balance of macronutrients and micronutrients.

For example, a balanced meal could look like:

- **Protein:** Grilled salmon (providing protein and healthy fats)

- **Vegetables:** Steamed broccoli and roasted sweet potatoes (providing vitamins, minerals, and fiber)
- **Grains:** Brown rice (providing complex carbohydrates and fiber)

To keep things interesting, try varying your proteins and grains throughout the week, incorporating both plant-based and animal-based options, and ensuring a variety of vegetables and fruits to meet different nutritional needs.

Sustainable Meal Planning: Reducing Food Waste and Saving Money

Beyond the personal health benefits, meal planning offers an incredible opportunity to contribute to sustainability by reducing food waste and minimizing environmental impact. The food system is responsible for a substantial portion of global greenhouse gas emissions, water usage, and land degradation. By planning meals with sustainability in mind, we can reduce our ecological footprint while also saving money and minimizing waste.

Reducing Food Waste

Food waste is a global issue that contributes to environmental degradation. Wasted food is often discarded in landfills, where it generates methane—one of the most potent greenhouse gases. The good news is that with careful planning and intentional practices, we can minimize this waste:

1. **Batch Cooking and Freezing:** When you prepare meals in large quantities, you can freeze leftovers, which will prevent them from being wasted. Soups,

stews, and casseroles freeze well and can be reheated later for another meal.
2. **Utilize Scraps:** Many vegetable scraps—such as onion skins, carrot tops, and potato peels—can be used to make broths or added to compost, reducing waste and enriching the soil.
3. **Repurpose Leftovers:** Repurposing leftovers into new meals is an excellent way to avoid throwing away food. For example, leftover rice can be used in a stir-fry, and extra vegetables can be added to a salad or frittata.

Saving Money

Meal planning can significantly cut grocery costs. By avoiding impulse buys and minimizing food waste, we can make the most of our grocery budget. Additionally, buying seasonal produce, purchasing in bulk, and focusing on plant-based proteins—such as lentils and beans—are cost-effective ways to save money while eating sustainably.

1. **Shop Smart:** Stick to a shopping list based on your meal plan, and avoid buying items you don't need. This helps avoid impulse purchases that can quickly add up.
2. **Buy in Bulk:** Purchasing grains, legumes, and nuts in bulk can save money and reduce packaging waste. These items have a long shelf life, making them easy to store and use across multiple meals.
3. **Choose Local and Seasonal Produce:** Seasonal fruits and vegetables are typically cheaper, fresher, and more nutrient-dense. Visiting a local farmers' market is a great way to support local agriculture while finding good deals.

Meal planning is a transformative practice that offers a wealth of benefits, not just for our personal health, but for the broader health of our planet. By approaching meal prepping with intention and care, we can make conscious decisions that promote better nutrition, minimize food waste, cut costs, and play a pivotal role in fostering a more sustainable and resilient food system. When we embrace sustainable meal planning, we're not only nourishing our bodies but also making a meaningful contribution to the planet's well-being. This holistic approach helps us live in alignment with our values—balancing personal well-being with environmental responsibility.

Through strategic planning and mindful food choices, we can cultivate a lifestyle that supports long-term health, reduces our ecological footprint, and encourages a more responsible relationship with the food system. By reducing food waste, choosing locally sourced and seasonal produce, and incorporating plant-based meals, we actively participate in protecting the environment while reaping the health benefits of a nutrient-dense diet. In this way, meal planning becomes a vital tool in creating a more balanced, nourishing, and sustainable way of living—one that nurtures both our bodies and the planet for generations to come.

Chapter 11

Navigating Plant-Based Eating

In today's world, there is a growing awareness about the profound impact our food choices have on both our personal health and the health of the planet. As we become more mindful of the environmental challenges we face and the links between diet and well-being, one dietary approach that has gained significant attention for its potential to improve health and foster sustainability is the plant-based diet. Plant-based eating is far more than a passing trend; it is a conscious decision to adopt a way of eating that prioritizes nutrient-dense foods derived from plants—such as vegetables, fruits, whole grains, legumes, nuts, and seeds—while minimizing or eliminating animal-based products.

This chapter delves into the numerous benefits of plant-based eating, both for your overall health and for the environment. From enhancing heart health to reducing the risk of chronic diseases, the benefits of plant-based foods are vast and well-documented. Equally important, plant-based diets have a significant role to play in mitigating climate change, conserving natural resources, and promoting biodiversity. In this chapter, we will explore these advantages in detail, showing how making more plant-based food choices can help you lead a healthier life while contributing to a more sustainable future.

We will also guide you through the practical steps of incorporating plant-based meals into your lifestyle, offering tips and strategies to make the transition seamless and enjoyable. Whether you are considering fully embracing a plant-based lifestyle or simply looking to introduce more plant-based options into your routine, this chapter will provide you with the knowledge and tools needed to make those changes effectively. Additionally, we will highlight the essential nutrients that plant-based eaters should focus on to ensure a well-rounded, nutritious diet, helping you to meet your dietary needs and achieve long-term health goals.

By the end of this chapter, you will have a comprehensive understanding of how plant-based eating can benefit your body, the environment, and your overall quality of life. We will offer practical advice, answer common questions, and share tips to help you navigate the plant-based journey with confidence, ensuring that you not only thrive in your dietary choices but also contribute to the greater good of the planet.

The Benefits of a Plant-Based Diet for Health and the Environment

Health Benefits of a Plant-Based Diet

A plant-based diet offers a wide range of health benefits, supported by numerous studies and health organizations worldwide. Below are some of the primary advantages:

1. **Improved Cardiovascular Health**
   One of the most well-documented benefits of plant-based eating is its positive impact on heart health. Plant-based foods—especially fruits, vegetables, whole grains, and legumes—are naturally rich in fiber, antioxidants, and healthy fats, all of which are known to improve cardiovascular function. The consumption of plant-based diets has been linked to lower blood pressure, reduced cholesterol levels, and a decreased risk of heart disease. Studies have found that those who follow plant-based diets have a lower

risk of developing hypertension, a leading cause of heart disease and stroke.

2. **Weight Management**
Plant-based eating can be beneficial for weight management. Fruits, vegetables, and whole grains are typically lower in calories but high in fiber, which helps promote feelings of fullness and reduces overall calorie intake. Plant-based diets are also rich in water, which adds bulk to the diet and aids in digestion. People who adopt plant-based eating patterns often report experiencing improved energy levels and a healthier body weight, as these diets promote fat loss while preserving lean muscle mass.

3. **Cancer Prevention**
A growing body of research suggests that plant-based diets may reduce the risk of certain cancers. The high fiber content of plant foods helps the body eliminate waste products and harmful toxins, potentially lowering the risk of colorectal cancer. Furthermore, fruits and vegetables contain a wide array of antioxidants and phytochemicals that have been shown to protect against cellular damage, which plays a role in the development of cancer. Studies also show that plant-based diets may help reduce the risk of breast, prostate, and other types of cancers.

4. **Diabetes Control and Prevention**
A plant-based diet can be highly effective in managing type 2 diabetes and preventing its onset. The abundance of fiber in plant-based foods helps regulate blood sugar levels, improving insulin sensitivity. Many plant-based foods, such as legumes, whole grains, and vegetables, have a low glycemic index, meaning they cause a slower and more stable rise in blood sugar, making them ideal for those managing diabetes. Research has shown that

individuals who follow plant-based diets often require less medication to control their diabetes and experience improved blood sugar levels and overall metabolic health.

5. **Improved Gut Health**
   The plant-based diet is rich in dietary fiber, which plays a critical role in gut health. Fiber feeds the beneficial bacteria in the digestive system, helping maintain a balanced gut microbiome. A healthy microbiome is linked to better digestion, improved immunity, and a reduced risk of gastrointestinal issues like constipation and bloating. The diversity of plant foods also supports a broader range of gut bacteria, which contributes to overall digestive wellness.

Environmental Benefits of a Plant-Based Diet

Beyond its health benefits, plant-based eating offers significant advantages for the environment. The global food system is responsible for a large portion of greenhouse gas emissions, deforestation, and water usage. Animal agriculture, in particular, is one of the leading contributors to environmental degradation. By shifting toward a plant-based diet, we can help reduce our environmental footprint. Here are some of the key environmental benefits of plant-based eating:

1. **Reduction in Greenhouse Gas Emissions**
   Animal agriculture is responsible for a substantial amount of greenhouse gas emissions, including methane and nitrous oxide. Methane, which is produced by livestock, is particularly potent—its global warming potential is over 25 times greater than carbon dioxide. Shifting away from animal-based products reduces the demand for meat and

dairy production, which, in turn, helps decrease these harmful emissions. Studies have shown that reducing meat consumption can lead to significant reductions in greenhouse gas emissions, contributing to efforts to combat climate change.

2. **Conservation of Water**
   The water footprint of animal products is far greater than that of plant-based foods. Producing a kilogram of beef requires thousands of liters of water for the animal's drinking water, feed crops, and processing. In contrast, growing plant-based foods like beans, lentils, and vegetables requires far less water. By adopting a plant-based diet, we can significantly reduce our water consumption, helping conserve this precious resource, which is becoming increasingly scarce in many parts of the world.

3. **Preservation of Biodiversity and Forests**
   Animal agriculture contributes to large-scale deforestation, particularly in regions like the Amazon Rainforest, where vast areas are cleared to create grazing land for cattle or to grow animal feed. This destruction of natural habitats leads to biodiversity loss, as countless species lose their homes. By reducing demand for meat and animal products, we can help preserve ecosystems and protect endangered species from habitat loss.

4. **Reduction in Land Use and Soil Degradation**
   Animal farming requires a substantial amount of land for grazing and growing feed crops. Converting large tracts of land for animal agriculture often leads to soil erosion and degradation. In contrast, plant-based foods typically require far less land and have a lower impact on soil health. By choosing plant-based options, we can help preserve arable land and promote sustainable farming practices.

How to Get Started with Plant-Based Meals

Transitioning to a plant-based diet doesn't have to be overwhelming. Whether you're going fully plant-based or just looking to reduce your animal product consumption, here are some practical steps to help you get started:

1. **Start Gradually**
   If you're new to plant-based eating, it's helpful to ease into it gradually. You don't have to make the switch overnight. Begin by incorporating more plant-based meals into your week, such as "Meatless Mondays" or swapping animal-based proteins for plant-based ones in familiar dishes. Over time, you can build up your repertoire of plant-based meals and gradually reduce your dependence on animal products.

2. **Explore New Ingredients**
   A plant-based diet opens up a whole new world of ingredients, many of which you might not be familiar with. Experiment with legumes (beans, lentils, chickpeas), whole grains (quinoa, farro, barley), plant-based milks (almond, soy, oat), and plant-based meat alternatives (tofu, tempeh, seitan). Don't be afraid to try new fruits and vegetables, and embrace different cooking techniques such as roasting, steaming, and sautéing to bring out the full flavors of plant-based foods.

3. **Plan Your Meals**
   One of the key components of transitioning to plant-based eating is meal planning. Preparing your meals ahead of time ensures that you always have nutritious, plant-based options available. Plan your meals around the plant-based proteins, grains, and

vegetables you enjoy, and try to include a variety of colorful ingredients to ensure that your meals are balanced and nutrient-dense.

4. **Educate Yourself**
   It's important to educate yourself about plant-based nutrition to ensure you're meeting all your dietary needs. While plant-based diets are typically rich in vitamins, minerals, and fiber, they may lack certain nutrients, such as vitamin B12, iron, and omega-3 fatty acids. Learn about these nutrients and how to incorporate plant-based sources, such as fortified foods, leafy greens, nuts, and seeds, into your diet.

5. **Seek Support**
   If you're feeling uncertain about transitioning to a plant-based diet, seek support from others who have made the shift. Join online communities, read plant-based cookbooks, or find local meet-ups or groups that support plant-based eating. Having a support system can make the transition easier and more enjoyable.

Key Nutrients for Plant-Based Eaters

While a plant-based diet offers an abundance of health benefits, it's essential to ensure you're getting all the necessary nutrients to stay healthy. Here are some key nutrients to focus on:

1. **Protein**
   Many people worry about getting enough protein on a plant-based diet. Fortunately, there are plenty of plant-based protein sources, including beans, lentils, chickpeas, tofu, tempeh, quinoa, edamame, nuts, and seeds. A diverse range of plant-based proteins will ensure that you meet your daily requirements.

2. **Vitamin B12**
Vitamin B12 is primarily found in animal products, so those following a plant-based diet should be mindful of this essential nutrient. It's important to include fortified foods, such as plant-based milks or nutritional yeast, or consider taking a B12 supplement to avoid deficiency.

3. **Iron**
Plant-based sources of iron include lentils, beans, tofu, quinoa, and spinach. However, the type of iron found in plants (non-heme iron) is not as easily absorbed by the body as the iron found in animal products (heme iron). To enhance absorption, pair iron-rich foods with vitamin C-rich foods, such as bell peppers, citrus fruits, or broccoli.

4. **Omega-3 Fatty Acids**
Omega-3 fatty acids are essential for heart health and cognitive function. While they are most commonly found in fatty fish, plant-based sources of omega-3s include flaxseeds, chia seeds, walnuts, and algae-based supplements.

5. **Calcium**
Calcium is vital for bone health, and while dairy products are a common source, plant-based options such as fortified plant milks, leafy greens, and tofu can provide ample amounts of calcium.

6. **Vitamin D**
Vitamin D is important for immune function and bone health. While sunlight is the best source of vitamin D, it may be beneficial for those on a plant-based diet to consume fortified foods or take a vitamin D supplement, especially during the winter months.

Navigating plant-based eating is not only an empowering journey, but a transformative one that offers a wealth of health benefits and a profound positive impact on the environment. By adopting the core principles of a plant-based diet—focusing on whole, nutrient-dense foods derived from plants—you can significantly enhance your health, energize your body, and contribute to a more sustainable future. Whether you're transitioning to a fully plant-based lifestyle or simply aiming to incorporate more plant-based meals into your weekly routine, the key to success lies in embracing variety, exploring new ingredients, and ensuring that your diet is both balanced and nutrient-rich.

Plant-based eating is a flexible and dynamic approach to nutrition that allows you to experiment with an exciting range of flavors, textures, and cooking methods. It's about discovering the vast array of vegetables, grains, legumes, nuts, seeds, and plant-based alternatives available to you, and creating meals that nourish your body while supporting your health goals. With the right knowledge and a little creativity, plant-based meals can be satisfying, delicious, and packed with the essential nutrients your body needs to thrive.

Incorporating plant-based foods into your diet is not only about removing animal products; it's about embracing a holistic approach that values sustainability, environmental conservation, and ethical eating. By shifting towards plant-based choices, you're making a direct contribution to reducing your carbon footprint, conserving water, and promoting the health of the planet —all while enhancing your own well-being. Whether you decide to adopt a plant-based diet full-time or integrate plant-based meals into your lifestyle, this journey is about making mindful choices that support both your health and the planet's future.

As you embark on this journey, remember that it's not about perfection, but progress. Experiment with new ingredients, try new recipes, and find joy in nourishing yourself with foods that not only benefit your body but also play a part in creating a more sustainable, ethical world. By focusing on variety, balanced nutrition, and mindful eating, you can easily navigate the world of plant-based eating and enjoy its many rewards—while feeling good about the positive impact you're making along the way.

Chapter 12

The Role of Meat and Animal Products in a Sustainable Diet

Meat and animal products have been central to human diets across cultures for centuries, serving not only as vital sources of nutrition but also as key elements of culinary traditions. These foods have shaped eating habits, providing essential nutrients and contributing to the rich diversity of flavors and textures in cuisines worldwide. However, as our understanding of health and sustainability evolves, there is a growing recognition of the need to reassess the role of animal-based foods in modern diets. Increasingly, the conversation revolves around how we can incorporate meat and animal products in a way that aligns with both our personal health goals and broader environmental concerns.

Today, many people continue to rely on meat and animal products for nourishment, as they offer an abundance of high-quality protein, essential vitamins, and minerals that are often difficult to obtain from plant-based sources alone. However, as dietary patterns evolve, so too does the call for a more responsible and mindful approach to consuming these foods. There is a growing focus on ensuring that animal products are consumed in a way that supports long-term health, minimizes food waste, and fosters optimal nutrition. Rather than advocating for the complete elimination of animal products, the goal is to explore how we can responsibly incorporate them into our diets in a balanced, sustainable manner.

This chapter aims to provide a deeper understanding of the role of meat and animal products in a sustainable diet. We will focus on the various nutritional benefits they offer, the potential challenges they present, and practical strategies for integrating them thoughtfully into a balanced diet. By doing so, we hope to offer a nuanced perspective that allows individuals to make informed choices about how and when to include animal products in their meals, ensuring that these foods support both their health and their broader sustainability goals.

The Nutritional Value of Meat and Animal Products

Meat and animal products are packed with essential nutrients that are often challenging to obtain from plant-based sources alone. These nutrients are integral to various bodily functions and are important for maintaining good health.

1. High-Quality Protein

One of the primary benefits of consuming meat and animal products is their high-quality protein content. Proteins are the building blocks of the body, essential for growth, tissue repair, immune function, and enzyme production. Animal-based proteins contain all nine essential amino acids required for optimal health, making them complete proteins. This is in contrast to many plant-based protein sources, which may lack one or more essential amino acids, requiring careful planning to ensure a balanced intake of protein.

Lean meats such as chicken, turkey, and fish provide high protein content with lower levels of fat, making them ideal sources for those seeking to meet their daily protein needs. Red meat, while still a good source of protein, is typically higher in saturated fat, which may be less beneficial when consumed in excess.

2. Iron and Zinc

Meat, particularly red meat, is an excellent source of heme iron, the type of iron most easily absorbed by the body. Iron is crucial for the production of hemoglobin in red blood cells, which transport oxygen throughout the body. While plant-based sources of iron (non-heme iron) exist, the absorption rate of non-heme iron is lower, making it more challenging for individuals, particularly those at higher risk of iron deficiency (such as pregnant women and young children), to meet their iron needs through plant sources alone.

In addition to iron, meat and animal products also provide a rich source of zinc, a mineral that plays a key role in immune function, cell division, and wound healing. Zinc from animal products is more bioavailable, meaning it is easier for the body to absorb and use compared to plant-based sources of zinc.

3. B Vitamins

Animal products, particularly meat, fish, eggs, and dairy, are rich in B vitamins, particularly B12, which is essential for nerve function, DNA synthesis, and red blood cell production. Vitamin B12 is almost exclusively found in animal-based foods, so those following a strictly plant-based diet need to consume fortified foods or take supplements to avoid deficiency. Additionally, meat and fish provide other B vitamins, such as niacin (B3), riboflavin (B2), and B6, all of which are important for energy production and maintaining healthy skin, eyes, and nerve function.

4. Omega-3 Fatty Acids

Fatty fish, such as salmon, mackerel, and sardines, are excellent sources of omega-3 fatty acids, which play a critical role in brain function, heart health, and inflammation reduction. Omega-3 fatty acids are essential fats that the body cannot produce on its own, meaning they must be obtained through diet. While plant-based sources of omega-3 (such as flaxseeds, chia seeds, and walnuts) provide alpha-linolenic acid (ALA), which the body can convert to the more bioactive forms of omega-3 (EPA and DHA), the conversion process is inefficient. Therefore, consuming fatty fish remains one of the most effective ways to obtain these essential fats.

5. Calcium and Vitamin D

Dairy products are a significant source of calcium, which is vital for bone health, muscle function, and nerve transmission. Calcium is also involved in the regulation of blood pressure and the functioning of enzymes. While calcium is available in some plant-based foods like fortified plant milks and leafy greens, dairy products remain one of the most reliable and bioavailable sources of this essential nutrient. Many dairy products are also fortified with vitamin D, which helps the body absorb calcium and supports immune health. For individuals who do not consume dairy, fortified plant-based alternatives or supplements may be necessary to ensure adequate intake of these nutrients.

The Challenges of Meat and Animal Products

While meat and animal products are rich in essential nutrients, it is important to recognize that their consumption comes with certain challenges that should not be overlooked. These challenges range from health concerns to ethical considerations, making it crucial to approach the inclusion of animal products in a sustainable diet with thoughtfulness and awareness. By considering these potential drawbacks—such as the impact of excessive saturated fat, the risks associated with processed meats, and the need for ethical sourcing —individuals can make more informed choices about how to incorporate these foods in a way that aligns with both their health goals and broader sustainability values. Thoughtful consumption allows for a balanced approach, maximizing the nutritional benefits while minimizing the negative effects on personal well-being, animal welfare.

1. Excessive Saturated Fat

One of the main concerns surrounding the consumption of animal products, especially red meat and processed meats, is the high content of saturated fat. Diets high in saturated fat have been linked to an increased risk of heart disease, stroke, and type 2 diabetes. Reducing the intake of saturated fat by choosing lean cuts of meat, limiting processed meats, and incorporating plant-based fats (such as those found in avocados, nuts, and olive oil) can help mitigate these health risks.

2. Processed Meats and Health Risks

Processed meats, such as sausages, bacon, hot dogs, and deli meats, have been classified by the World Health Organization (WHO) as carcinogenic to humans, with studies showing a link between their consumption and an increased risk of colorectal cancer. These meats often contain preservatives and additives like nitrates, which can form harmful compounds when consumed in excess. Limiting processed meats and focusing on fresh, minimally processed animal products is a healthier choice for those who include meat in their diet.

3. Ethical Considerations

For some individuals, the ethical concerns surrounding meat and animal product consumption are a key factor in their decision to reduce or eliminate these foods from their diets. The treatment of animals in factory farming operations, concerns over animal welfare, and the ethical implications of consuming animal products have sparked widespread debates. Many consumers are opting for ethically sourced, free-range, or grass-fed meat options that prioritize animal welfare and more humane farming practices.

4. Foodborne Illnesses and Safety

Raw or undercooked meat, particularly poultry, pork, and beef, can be a source of foodborne illnesses like Salmonella, E. coli, and Listeria. To reduce the risk of foodborne illness, it is important to handle, store, and cook meat products properly. This includes following food safety guidelines such as maintaining proper refrigeration, cooking meat to the recommended temperature, and avoiding cross-contamination.

How to Incorporate Meat and Animal Products Responsibly

To integrate meat and animal products into a sustainable and health-conscious diet, it is essential to approach consumption mindfully. Here are some tips for including these foods while maintaining a balanced and responsible diet:

1. Prioritize Lean and Whole Animal Products

When consuming meat, it's important to prioritize lean cuts of meat, such as chicken breast, turkey, and lean cuts of beef and pork. These cuts have lower levels of saturated fat, making them a healthier choice. Additionally, focusing on whole animal products such as unprocessed meats, eggs, and dairy, rather than processed options, can help reduce health risks.

2. Practice Portion Control

Moderation is key when it comes to meat consumption. Rather than making meat the centerpiece of every meal, aim to make it a smaller part of a balanced plate. Incorporating more plant-based foods, such as vegetables, grains, legumes, and legumes, can help reduce your overall intake of animal products while still ensuring you receive a variety of nutrients.

3. Choose Sustainable and Ethical Sourcing

For those who continue to include animal products in their diet, choosing sustainably sourced, ethical options is important. Look for meat and dairy products that are certified organic, grass-fed, or free-range, as these typically come from farms with more humane practices and a reduced environmental footprint.

4. Rotate Animal Proteins with Plant-Based Alternatives

A flexible approach to protein consumption can involve rotating animal products with plant-based proteins, such as beans, lentils, tofu, tempeh, and quinoa. By including a variety of protein sources in your diet, you can achieve balanced nutrition while supporting a more sustainable food system.

Meat and animal products continue to play a vital role in many people's diets by providing high-quality protein, essential vitamins, and minerals. These foods are key sources of nutrients that support various bodily functions, such as muscle repair, immune health, and cognitive function. However, it is essential to approach their consumption thoughtfully, weighing both the health benefits and potential drawbacks.

Focusing on lean, minimally processed cuts of meat and practicing portion control can help mitigate the risks associated with high saturated fat intake, while ensuring that the nutritional benefits of animal products are maximized. By choosing high-quality, ethically raised animal products, individuals can make healthier and more responsible choices that align with their dietary needs. Prioritizing moderation, as well as incorporating a variety of protein sources into the diet, ensures that animal products are enjoyed in a balanced way. This approach allows for the continued enjoyment of meat and animal-based foods while fostering a nutritious and well-rounded diet.

Chapter 13

Cooking for Health and the Planet

In today's fast-paced world, cooking has evolved beyond its basic role of providing nourishment—it has become an opportunity to make a meaningful and lasting impact on both our health and the environment. The choices we make in the kitchen, from the ingredients we select to the methods we employ, directly influence not only our well-being but also the ecological footprint we leave behind. Each meal we prepare offers a chance to embrace healthier, more sustainable practices that benefit both ourselves and the planet.

This chapter will take you on a journey through eco-friendly kitchen practices, exploring energy-saving tips, waste reduction strategies, and the importance of choosing ingredients that align with a sustainable food system. We'll also delve into healthy cooking methods—such as steaming, roasting, and sauteing—that preserve the nutritional integrity of your food while reducing the need for excess fats or unhealthy additives. Finally, we'll explore how to create delicious, balanced meals by finding the right harmony between animal and plant-based ingredients.

By adopting sustainable cooking practices, you can not only enhance the flavors and nutritional value of your meals but also contribute to a more responsible and resilient food system. Cooking thoughtfully is a powerful tool that enables you to make choices that promote health, protect the environment, and create a more sustainable future for generations to come. Whether you're a seasoned cook or a beginner, the insights and techniques shared in this chapter will empower you to cook with intention, making every meal a step toward a healthier and more sustainable lifestyle.

Eco-Friendly Kitchen Practices: Energy-Saving Tips and Waste Reduction

The kitchen is one of the most energy-intensive areas of the home. From heating stoves to running dishwashers, every step in food preparation has an environmental cost. Fortunately, by implementing eco-friendly kitchen practices, you can significantly reduce energy usage, minimize food waste, and lower your overall carbon footprint.

1. Reduce Energy Consumption

One of the simplest ways to make your cooking more eco-friendly is to reduce energy consumption in the kitchen. This not only helps save resources but can also reduce your utility bills.

- **Use Energy-Efficient Appliances:** Choose appliances that are energy-efficient, such as induction cooktops, energy-efficient ovens, and refrigerators with a high energy rating. Induction cooktops, for example, are known to be faster and more energy-efficient than traditional electric or gas stoves.
- **Cook in Batches:** Preparing multiple meals or large batches of food at once can save both time and energy. It reduces the need to use the oven or stove frequently, which can lead to significant energy savings in the long run. Additionally, cooking larger

quantities allows you to use leftovers throughout the week, reducing food waste.

- **Opt for Small Appliances:** Using a toaster oven or slow cooker can be more energy-efficient than heating up a large oven. A slow cooker or pressure cooker uses less energy and is an ideal choice for long cooking processes like stews or soups.
- **Cook with Lids On:** Cooking with lids on pots or pans helps retain heat and reduces cooking time, which in turn saves energy. Keeping your kitchen well-insulated and sealing your pots tightly can maximize efficiency during cooking.

2. Reduce Food Waste

Food waste is a major environmental issue, and it's essential to minimize waste wherever possible. The U.S. alone wastes approximately 40% of its food each year, which contributes to greenhouse gas emissions and unnecessarily depletes resources. Here are some strategies to reduce food waste in the kitchen:

- **Plan Meals and Shop Smart:** Meal planning is a key practice in reducing food waste. By planning your meals for the week, you can purchase only what you need, ensuring that ingredients aren't wasted. It's also important to check your pantry and fridge regularly to use up ingredients that are nearing their expiration dates.
- **Proper Food Storage:** Store fruits, vegetables, and other perishables properly to extend their shelf life. For instance, keeping leafy greens in a moisture-proof container can help them stay fresh longer. Additionally, freezing leftovers or surplus ingredients like berries, vegetables, or meat can extend their usability and prevent them from spoiling.

- **Compost Scraps:** Composting food scraps is an excellent way to divert waste from landfills and enrich soil for gardening. Vegetable peels, coffee grounds, eggshells, and other organic waste can all be composted, reducing landfill waste and supporting sustainable practices.
- **Repurpose Leftovers:** Get creative with your leftovers by transforming them into new meals. For instance, yesterday's roasted vegetables can become today's salad topping, and stale bread can be turned into croutons. This minimizes waste and ensures that nothing goes to waste.

3. Eco-Friendly Cleaning

Using eco-friendly cleaning products in your kitchen is another important step in reducing your environmental footprint. Opt for biodegradable dish soaps, all-purpose cleaners, and non-toxic products that don't harm the environment. Reusable dish cloths, sponges, and cleaning towels can replace paper products, reducing waste.

Healthy Cooking Methods: Steaming, Roasting, and Sauteing

The way we cook our food plays a crucial role in preserving its nutrients and enhancing its health benefits. Cooking methods such as steaming, roasting, and sauteing are not only healthier options but also help maintain the integrity of the ingredients while minimizing the use of excessive fats or oils.

1. Steaming: Retaining Nutrients

Steaming is one of the healthiest cooking methods as it retains most of the nutrients in vegetables, grains, and fish. When you steam food, it is cooked by hot steam, which gently cooks the ingredients while preserving their vitamins and minerals that may otherwise be lost through boiling or frying.

- **Benefits of Steaming:**
    - Retains vitamins and minerals, particularly water-soluble ones like Vitamin C and folate, which are often lost in boiling or frying.
    - Helps reduce the need for additional fats, making it an ideal method for low-calorie, heart-healthy meals.
    - Steaming can enhance the natural flavor of the food, making it more enjoyable without adding extra seasonings or fats.
- **Steaming Tips:**
    - Use a steamer basket to cook vegetables or fish, ensuring that the food doesn't come into direct contact with water. You can also use a microwave-safe bowl with a lid for steaming small portions.
    - For added flavor, steam your vegetables with herbs or lemon slices to infuse a fresh taste without the need for excess salt or oil.

2. Roasting: Enhancing Flavor Without Excessive Fats

Roasting is another healthy cooking method that brings out the natural sweetness and richness of vegetables, meats, and other ingredients. By roasting food in the oven, you can create a crispy texture while retaining most of the nutrients.

- **Benefits of Roasting:**
    - Roasting vegetables at high temperatures caramelizes their natural sugars, enhancing their flavor without the need for extra fats or sugars.
    - This method is perfect for root vegetables like sweet potatoes, carrots, and beets, which become more tender and flavorful when roasted.
    - Roasting meats like chicken or fish can result in a crispy, golden exterior while keeping the interior moist and tender.
- **Roasting Tips:**
    - Avoid overuse of oils by using a light mist of olive oil or choosing a roasting pan with a non-stick surface.
    - For a healthier meal, pair roasted vegetables with a small amount of lean protein, such as chicken or plant-based proteins like tofu or tempeh.
    - Experiment with seasonings like garlic, rosemary, thyme, and paprika to add depth of flavor without excess fat or salt.

3. Sauteing: Quick and Flavorful

Sauteing is a quick cooking method that involves cooking food over medium-high heat in a small amount of fat, such as olive oil or coconut oil. This method is

great for vegetables, grains, and lean meats, as it preserves their texture while locking in flavors.
- **Benefits of Sauteing:**
    - Sauteing allows for quick cooking, which can help retain nutrients that might be lost during prolonged cooking times.
    - It uses less oil than frying, making it a healthier option for preparing vegetables and proteins.
    - You can experiment with a wide variety of ingredients and spices to create rich, flavorful meals in a short amount of time.
- **Sauteing Tips:**
    - Use a non-stick skillet to minimize the need for excess oil.
    - Choose healthy oils like olive oil or avocado oil, which are rich in heart-healthy monounsaturated fats.
    - To add more flavor, try sauteing vegetables with garlic, onions, or fresh herbs, and finish the dish with a splash of lemon or balsamic vinegar for extra brightness.

How to Create Delicious Meals with a Balance Between Animal and Non-Animal Products

One of the key principles of a sustainable and healthy diet is balance. While plant-based eating has many environmental and health benefits, incorporating moderate amounts of responsibly sourced animal products can also be part of a healthy diet. Finding the right balance between animal and non-animal products ensures that you get the variety of nutrients your body needs while still supporting a sustainable food system.

1. Prioritize Plant-Based Ingredients

When planning meals, make plants the star of the plate. Focus on filling half your plate with vegetables, whole grains, legumes, nuts, and seeds. These foods provide the essential nutrients, fiber, and antioxidants that are key to a healthy, balanced diet.

2. Choose Sustainable Animal Products

When including animal products in your meals, opt for sustainably sourced options. Look for grass-fed, pasture-raised, and hormone-free meats, as well as wild-caught fish or certified organic poultry. These options tend to have a smaller environmental impact and provide higher-quality nutrition compared to conventionally raised animal products.

3. Portion Control with Animal Products

If you choose to include animal products in your meals, aim for smaller portions and use them as a complement to plant-based foods rather than the main event. For example, pair a small portion of grilled chicken with a hearty salad or mix lean beef with plenty of vegetables in a stir-fry.

4. Experiment with Plant-Based Alternatives

Incorporate plant-based alternatives to animal products when possible. Tofu, tempeh, lentils, beans, and plant-based dairy products are excellent substitutes that can be used to create satisfying meals. These alternatives are not only great for your health, but they also reduce the environmental impact of your diet.

As a result, cooking for health and the planet is not just a practice, but a mindset that empowers you to make meaningful, sustainable choices every time you step into the kitchen. It's a way of eating that goes beyond just feeding yourself—it's about nurturing your body while simultaneously taking care of the planet. Each decision, from the ingredients you choose to the cooking methods you use, holds the power to contribute positively to both your personal well-being and the larger environment.

By adopting energy-saving practices in the kitchen, you're not only reducing your energy bill but also minimizing the carbon footprint of your cooking. Simple changes like using energy-efficient appliances, cooking in batches, or reducing the use of single-use items can lead to substantial energy savings. Likewise, reducing food waste through careful planning and proper food storage reduces the environmental burden of producing food that is never consumed. When we waste less food, we help conserve the precious resources—land, water, and energy—that went into producing it.

Choosing healthier cooking methods, such as steaming, roasting, and sauteing, allows you to preserve the natural nutrients in your food while minimizing the need for excess fats or oils. This focus on health-conscious cooking methods not only supports your physical health but also reflects a commitment to mindful consumption—ensuring that every meal you prepare is both nourishing and planet-friendly. By making these small changes in how we cook, we're supporting a larger shift toward a food system that values sustainability, nutritional integrity, and ethical sourcing.

Incorporating a balance of plant-based and animal-based foods in your diet is another crucial step toward sustainability. By choosing high-quality, responsibly sourced animal products and focusing on plant-based ingredients, you can optimize both your health and the environment. This balanced approach helps reduce the environmental impact of animal agriculture—such as greenhouse gas emissions and water usage—while providing the essential nutrients your body needs. It's not about completely eliminating animal products, but rather about finding a sustainable balance that works for you and supports a more ethical, conscious food system.

The journey to cooking for health and sustainability is one of progress, not perfection. Every choice you make, no matter how small, has a ripple effect. Whether it's incorporating more plant-based meals, using less plastic, or finding new ways to reduce food waste, each step leads you closer to a healthier, more sustainable way of living. With every meal, you are voting with your fork, choosing a path that reflects your values and desires for a better world. As you continue on this journey, remember that it's not about achieving perfection—it's about the daily decisions and small changes that collectively make a big difference for your health and the planet.

Chapter 14

Sustainable Eating on a Budget

Eating sustainably doesn't have to come with a hefty price tag. In fact, with a mindful approach, you can prioritize both your health and the environment without straining your finances. Sustainable eating is often seen as expensive, especially when it comes to purchasing organic foods, buying fresh, local produce, or opting for specialty items. However, this perception can be easily challenged with some smart planning and cost-effective strategies that allow you to enjoy a nourishing and eco-friendly diet without breaking the bank.

This chapter will guide you through practical ways to eat healthily and sustainably while being mindful of your budget. We'll delve into strategies for sourcing organic and locally grown produce at a lower cost, explore ways to minimize food waste, and offer creative meal ideas that emphasize nutritional value without overspending. You'll learn how to make small, thoughtful adjustments to your shopping habits, meal planning, and food preparation that can lead to significant savings and a more sustainable lifestyle.

By the end of this chapter, you'll have a comprehensive understanding of how to build a sustainable, budget-friendly diet that not only supports your well-being but also contributes positively to the planet. Whether you're on a tight budget or simply looking to make more conscious choices at the grocery store, these practical tips will empower you to take charge of your health and make environmentally responsible decisions—without the financial stress.

How to Eat Healthily and Sustainably Without Breaking the Bank

Sustainable eating is about making intentional, mindful choices that prioritize both your long-term health and the health of the planet. It's a way of eating that seeks to balance personal nutrition with environmental responsibility. This approach goes beyond simply choosing organic or locally sourced foods—it involves actively reducing reliance on highly processed, packaged, and resource-intensive foods, while focusing on whole, plant-based options that are nourishing for both the body and the earth. Fresh fruits, vegetables, whole grains, legumes, nuts, seeds, and plant-based proteins provide essential nutrients and offer a much lower environmental footprint compared to conventional animal products and processed foods.

While it's true that some sustainable products may come with a higher upfront cost, there are many ways to incorporate sustainable eating into your life without breaking the bank. It's important to remember that the true cost of food isn't just about the price tag at the checkout. When we factor in long-term health benefits, reduced environmental damage, and the promotion of a more equitable food system, sustainable eating often proves to be more economical in the grand scheme.

By adopting strategies like shopping seasonally, buying in bulk, cooking from scratch, and embracing plant-based meals, you can enjoy healthy, affordable, and sustainable meals. Additionally, being strategic with meal planning and reducing food waste allows you to make the most of your food purchases, ensuring that you maximize every ingredient's potential. Sustainable eating is about finding the right balance between cost, nutrition, and environmental impact, and with a few key adjustments, you can align your food choices with your values, all while staying within your budget.

- **Embrace Plant-Based Eating**
  One of the most effective ways to reduce food costs while eating sustainably is by incorporating more plant-based foods into your meals. Plant-based proteins—such as beans, lentils, tofu, and chickpeas—are often more affordable than animal proteins like meat and dairy, and they are also better for the environment. Beans and lentils, for example, are rich in protein and fiber and can be purchased in bulk at a lower cost. By building your meals around these ingredients, you can significantly reduce your grocery bills while eating healthily.

- **Plan Your Meals in Advance**
  Meal planning is a simple yet powerful tool for saving money and ensuring you eat sustainably. When you plan your meals in advance, you can make sure you're purchasing only the ingredients you need, reducing the likelihood of food waste. Creating a weekly meal plan also gives you the opportunity to focus on seasonal produce, which is often cheaper and more abundant. By sticking to a shopping list based on your meal plan, you can avoid impulse buys and make healthier, more sustainable choices at the grocery store.

- **Buy in Bulk**
  Buying staples like grains, legumes, and nuts in bulk is an excellent way to save money while supporting sustainable eating. Bulk foods typically cost less per unit than packaged products and come with less waste. Many grocery stores now offer bulk bins for items such as rice, oats, quinoa, lentils, and beans. You can purchase only the amount you need, which

helps reduce food waste and saves money in the long run.

- **Focus on Frozen and Canned Produce**
  Fresh produce can sometimes be expensive, especially when it's out of season. However, frozen and canned fruits and vegetables are often more affordable, have a longer shelf life, and retain much of their nutritional value. Stocking up on frozen vegetables and fruits allows you to enjoy seasonal produce year-round without the high cost. Just be sure to choose options without added sugars, salt, or preservatives. Canned beans, tomatoes, and other vegetables are also cost-effective, convenient, and environmentally friendly choices.

- **Shop at Farmers' Markets or Join a CSA**
  Farmers' markets and community-supported agriculture (CSA) programs offer a direct way to support local, sustainable agriculture. Often, produce sold at these markets is more affordable than what you would find at larger supermarkets, especially when purchased in bulk or at the end of the market day. Many farmers' markets offer discounts or specials, so it's worth exploring these options. CSAs allow you to purchase a share of a local farm's produce, often at a lower cost than buying individual items at the store. Additionally, buying directly from farmers helps support local agriculture and reduces the environmental impact of long-distance food transport.

Cost-Effective Strategies for Sourcing Organic and Local Produce

Eating organic and locally sourced foods is a great way to support sustainability, but it can be difficult to do so on a tight budget. However, there are strategies to make organic and local foods more affordable.

- **Prioritize the Dirty Dozen and Clean Fifteen**
  If you're concerned about the cost of organic produce, start by focusing on the "Dirty Dozen"—the twelve fruits and vegetables most contaminated by pesticides—and opt for organic versions of these items. For the other fruits and vegetables, you can stick to conventional produce or prioritize the "Clean Fifteen," which includes items that tend to have lower pesticide residues. The Environmental Working Group (EWG) provides an annual guide to these lists, helping you make informed choices about which organic products are worth the investment.

- **Buy in Season**
  Seasonal produce is often more affordable, fresher, and more abundant than out-of-season fruits and vegetables. By shopping for fruits and vegetables that are in season, you not only save money but also reduce your environmental footprint by supporting crops that are grown locally. For example, root vegetables like carrots and potatoes are usually cheaper in the fall and winter, while summer fruits like berries and tomatoes are best purchased during their peak season. Planning meals around what's in season can help you stick to a budget and enjoy the best flavors nature has to offer.

- **Grow Your Own Food**
  If you have the space and time, growing your own fruits and vegetables is one of the most cost-effective ways to eat sustainably. Even if you only have a small balcony or windowsill, you can grow herbs, leafy greens, tomatoes, and other small vegetables. Starting with easy-to-grow plants like lettuce, spinach, or herbs like basil and parsley can provide

fresh ingredients for your meals throughout the season, reducing the need for store-bought produce. Community gardens are another great option for those who may not have access to land but want to grow their own food.

- **Use Store Loyalty Programs and Coupons**
  Many supermarkets offer loyalty programs and digital coupons that can help you save money on organic and local produce. By signing up for store newsletters and loyalty cards, you can gain access to exclusive discounts, promotional offers, and rewards. Additionally, there are a growing number of apps and websites dedicated to finding and sharing grocery store discounts, which can help you score savings on organic items and other sustainably produced foods.

Creative Meal Ideas for Frugal, Nutritious Eating

Eating sustainably on a budget doesn't mean sacrificing flavor or nutrition. With a little creativity, you can make delicious and nutritious meals using affordable, plant-based ingredients. Here are a few ideas to get you started:

- **Vegetable Stir-Fry**
  Stir-fries are a quick, budget-friendly way to use up leftover vegetables and grains. By combining affordable vegetables like carrots, broccoli, bell peppers, and onions with a simple sauce made from soy sauce, garlic, and a dash of sesame oil, you can create a healthy, flavorful dish that can be served over rice or noodles. Add a plant-based protein like tofu or tempeh to increase the protein content.

- **Lentil Soup**
  Lentils are an incredibly inexpensive source of

protein and fiber, making them a staple in any frugal, sustainable kitchen. A hearty lentil soup can be made with ingredients you likely already have on hand, such as carrots, celery, onions, garlic, and canned tomatoes. Lentils cook quickly, and you can easily freeze leftovers for future meals. Add greens like spinach or kale for an extra nutrient boost.

- **Chickpea Salad**
  Chickpeas are versatile, affordable, and packed with protein. You can use canned or dried chickpeas to create a simple salad with chopped vegetables like cucumbers, tomatoes, and red onions, along with a lemon-tahini dressing. This dish is not only nutritious but also filling, making it a great option for meal prepping or packing lunches.

- **Rice and Beans**
  Rice and beans are the quintessential budget-friendly meal that provides both protein and fiber. A simple dish of brown rice and black beans can be spiced with cumin, chili powder, garlic, and onions for a satisfying meal. Top with avocado, salsa, and cilantro for added flavor and nutrients. You can also swap in other beans such as kidney beans or pinto beans depending on your preferences and what's on sale.

- **Vegetable Curry**
  Curries are a fantastic way to use up a variety of vegetables while infusing your meals with rich, flavorful spices. A vegetable curry made with potatoes, carrots, peas, and cauliflower, along with coconut milk and curry spices, is an affordable yet satisfying meal. Serve it over brown rice or quinoa to complete the meal.

Sustainable eating on a budget is not only possible, but it can also be both enjoyable and rewarding with the right approach. By embracing plant-based meals, thoughtful meal planning, and implementing cost-effective strategies such as buying in bulk, shopping seasonally, and seeking out local produce, you can maintain a healthy, eco-friendly diet without stretching your budget. The key lies in being resourceful and creative—whether it's sourcing affordable organic options, growing your own food, or making the most of versatile, nutritious ingredients. By adopting these strategies, you'll not only nourish your body and save money, but you'll also reduce your environmental impact, all while fostering a more sustainable food system. The result is a diet that benefits both your health and the planet, proving that conscious choices can lead to lasting, positive changes for both your lifestyle and the world around you.

Chapter 15

Seasonal Eating: A Guide to Eating with the Seasons

Eating with the seasons is an ancient tradition that has been deeply rooted in human culture for centuries, long before the advent of supermarkets and global food supply chains. In the past, people's diets were directly influenced by what could be grown locally and what was available at different times of the year. Today, with rising concerns over sustainability, climate change, and personal health, seasonal eating is experiencing a powerful resurgence as a pivotal practice for cultivating healthier, more environmentally conscious lifestyles. By choosing foods that are in season, we not only enjoy the freshest and most flavorful produce, but we also contribute to a more sustainable food system, support local farmers, and reduce our environmental impact.

In this chapter, we will delve into the many compelling benefits of eating in-season produce. By embracing the rhythm of the seasons, we can reconnect with nature's cycles and make mindful food choices that are not only good for our health but also beneficial for the planet. We will explore how seasonal eating supports local economies, strengthens community ties, and promotes biodiversity. Additionally, we will share practical tips on how to navigate seasonal produce, what to buy in each season, and how to preserve excess produce to reduce food waste and ensure that the vibrant flavors of each season can be enjoyed year-round.

By understanding the importance of eating seasonally, you can take meaningful steps toward creating a more sustainable lifestyle. This chapter will empower you with the knowledge and tools you need to embrace seasonal eating, making it a natural and enjoyable part of your everyday routine. Whether you're a seasoned advocate of seasonal eating or just beginning to explore the benefits, this guide will offer practical insights and inspiration to help you make the most of nature's bounty, all while nurturing both your body and the planet.

The Benefits of Eating In-Season Produce

- **Improved Taste and Quality**

One of the most immediate and rewarding benefits of eating seasonal produce is the superior taste and quality of fruits and vegetables that are in season. Unlike out-of-season produce that is often harvested prematurely to survive long storage times and transportation, seasonal produce is allowed to ripen naturally in its ideal growing conditions, absorbing nutrients from the soil and reaching its full flavor potential. This results in fruits and vegetables with a more vibrant, robust, and complex flavor profile. Seasonal produce is picked at the peak of its ripeness, ensuring a level of taste and freshness that is often unmatched by its out-of-season counterparts.

Additionally, because seasonal produce doesn't require extended shipping or refrigeration, it typically arrives at your table fresher and with fewer chemical treatments, allowing it to retain its natural nutrients. As a result, seasonal fruits and vegetables are not only tastier, but they are also more nutrient-dense. For instance, a tomato harvested in the height of summer, when it's naturally exposed to the sun, will have significantly more flavor and sweetness than one grown in a greenhouse or imported from distant regions during the winter months, where it may be harvested while still green and forced to ripen artificially. The difference in taste is striking—fresh, in-season tomatoes burst with juiciness and complexity, while out-of-season tomatoes often lack the same depth and richness.

In short, eating with the seasons means enjoying the freshest, most flavorful produce that nature has to offer, allowing you to experience the full range of flavors and textures that truly seasonal foods can provide.

- **Nutritional Value**

In-season produce tends to be at its peak nutritional value. Freshly picked fruits and vegetables are packed with vitamins, minerals, and antioxidants that can degrade over time, especially when stored for long periods or shipped across long distances. The shorter the time between harvest and consumption, the better the nutritional content. For example, spinach picked in the spring has more vitamin C and folate than spinach that's been stored in a warehouse or shipped from another country. Seasonal eating ensures that you're consuming produce at its most nutrient-dense, which can lead to better health outcomes over time.

- **Cost-Effectiveness**

Seasonal produce is often more affordable than out-of-season produce. When fruits and vegetables are in abundance, the price generally drops due to the larger supply. Farmers are able to grow more crops when they're naturally in season, and this increased supply lowers the cost for consumers. Out-of-season produce, on the other hand, is typically more expensive due to the higher costs of transportation, energy, and storage. By purchasing in-season produce, you're more likely to find affordable options that fit within your budget while still providing high-quality, fresh food.

- **Supporting Local Farmers and Reducing Your Carbon Footprint**

Eating seasonally means supporting local farmers who grow crops that thrive in your region's climate. When you buy locally grown, in-season produce, you're directly contributing to the local economy and ensuring that farmers can continue to grow food that sustains their livelihoods. Moreover, purchasing seasonal food reduces the need for transportation and refrigeration, which in turn decreases carbon emissions. When produce is grown closer to home, it doesn't need to travel long distances by air, land, or sea, which reduces its overall environmental impact. Seasonal eating is an effective way to lower your carbon footprint and contribute to more sustainable food systems.

- **Reducing Food Waste**

By eating with the seasons, you also help minimize food waste. In-season produce is harvested in greater quantities and can be preserved for future use, whether through freezing, canning, or drying. This not only ensures that the bounty of each season isn't wasted but also provides you with options to enjoy seasonal flavors throughout the year. Furthermore, seasonal produce is often harvested at the ideal time, meaning it is less likely to spoil quickly compared to out-of-season options, which may have been stored for extended periods before reaching your plate.

How Seasonal Eating Supports Local Farmers and Reduces Your Carbon Footprint

- **Strengthening Local Economies**

When you choose to eat foods that are in-season and grown locally, you are supporting farmers in your community. Many small-scale farmers depend on the sale of seasonal produce to sustain their businesses, and by choosing to buy from them, you help ensure their success. Furthermore, supporting local food systems helps promote agricultural diversity, as farmers are more likely to grow a variety of crops that are suited to the local climate. This reduces the dependency on large agribusinesses and contributes to more resilient, sustainable farming practices.

In addition to benefiting farmers, seasonal eating encourages the growth of farmers' markets, co-ops, and community-supported agriculture (CSA) programs. These programs create closer connections between consumers and producers, allowing people to learn more about where their food comes from and how it is grown. These closer relationships often result in more transparency in the food system, which builds trust and promotes a more ethical and sustainable food economy.

- **Lower Carbon Footprint**

A significant environmental benefit of seasonal eating is the reduction in carbon emissions. The longer the supply chain for a particular food, the greater the carbon footprint. When foods are grown out of season, they are typically transported from distant locations via planes, trucks, or ships, which requires significant energy and fossil fuels. According to studies, food transportation contributes a large portion of a meal's overall carbon footprint, particularly for foods that are grown far from where they are consumed.

By eating locally grown, in-season foods, we drastically reduce the distance that food travels, minimizing the associated carbon emissions. Additionally, when food is harvested and consumed at the peak of the growing season, it requires less artificial refrigeration and packaging, both of which contribute to the environmental impact of food transportation.

What to Buy Each Season and How to Preserve Excess Produce

Eating seasonally requires knowledge of what produce is in season at different times of the year. Below is a guide to help you know what to buy during each season, as well as tips on how to preserve excess produce for later use.

Spring

Spring is a time of renewal, and the market is filled with vibrant, tender vegetables and fruits that mark the end of winter. Some of the most common spring produce includes:

- **Asparagus** : Fresh, tender stalks that are rich in vitamins A, C, and K.
- **Spinach** : Full of iron, fiber, and antioxidants, spinach is a springtime favorite.
- **Peas** : Sweet and crisp, peas are high in protein and fiber.
- **Strawberries** : One of the first fruits to ripen, offering a burst of sweetness and vitamin C.

Preservation Tips : Many spring vegetables like peas and spinach can be frozen or blanched to preserve their freshness. You can also make strawberry jam or preserve them in syrup to enjoy throughout the year.

Summer

Summer is abundant with a variety of fruits and vegetables at their peak. Some of the most popular summer produce includes:

- **Tomatoes** : Rich in lycopene, tomatoes are perfect for sauces, salads, and fresh salsas.
- **Cucumbers** : Refreshing and hydrating, cucumbers are great for summer salads.
- **Zucchini** : A versatile vegetable, zucchini can be grilled, roasted, or added to stir-fries.
- **Berries** : Blueberries, raspberries, and blackberries are at their best in the summer and are packed with antioxidants.

Preservation Tips : Summer fruits like tomatoes and berries can be canned, frozen, or made into preserves. Zucchini can be shredded and frozen for later use in baking or casseroles.

Fall

Fall is harvest time, and markets are filled with hearty, filling produce that keeps us satisfied as the weather turns cooler. Some fall favorites include:

- **Pumpkin** : High in fiber and vitamin A, pumpkin can be roasted, pureed, or used in soups and pies.
- **Apples** : Crisp, sweet apples are perfect for snacking, baking, or making applesauce.

- **Squash** : Varieties like butternut and acorn squash are nutrient-rich and perfect for roasting.
- **Brussels sprouts** : These tiny cabbages are rich in vitamin C and fiber.

Preservation Tips : Fall produce like squash and pumpkin can be stored in a cool, dry place for several months. Apples can be stored in the fridge or canned for later use.

Winter

Winter is a time for root vegetables, hardy greens, and citrus fruits that thrive in colder temperatures. Some common winter produce includes:

- **Carrots** : Sweet and versatile, carrots are high in vitamin A.
- **Kale** : Packed with nutrients like calcium and vitamin K, kale thrives in the winter.
- **Citrus** : Oranges, grapefruits, and lemons are packed with vitamin C and help boost the immune system during cold weather.
- **Sweet potatoes** : Rich in beta-carotene, fiber, and potassium, sweet potatoes are perfect for hearty meals.

Preservation Tips : Winter root vegetables can be stored in the fridge or root cellar for several weeks. Citrus can be juiced or preserved into marmalade for later use.

Eating with the seasons is a simple yet profoundly impactful choice that can transform the way you approach food, benefiting both your health and the planet. By choosing seasonal produce, you're not only enjoying fresher, more flavorful foods but also actively reducing your environmental footprint. Seasonal foods require less transportation and fewer artificial inputs, such as refrigeration and preservatives, which significantly cuts down on their carbon footprint. Supporting local farmers by purchasing in-season produce strengthens regional food systems, helping small-scale agriculture thrive and promoting a more resilient, sustainable food economy.

In addition to its environmental and ethical advantages, seasonal eating also encourages you to expand your culinary horizons. Each season offers a unique array of fruits and vegetables that you may not have considered, increasing the diversity of your diet and introducing you to new flavors, textures, and nutrients. By embracing seasonal produce, you not only enjoy a greater variety of nutrients—such as vitamins, minerals, and antioxidants—but you also foster a more balanced, wholesome diet. Seasonal eating is a gateway to eating more mindfully, reconnecting with nature's rhythms, and supporting biodiversity by promoting the cultivation of a wide range of crops that are well-suited to the climate and growing conditions of your region.

By incorporating the tips and principles outlined in this chapter, you can create a sustainable eating routine that nourishes both your body and the planet. Whether you're cooking simple, everyday meals or experimenting with new ingredients, seasonal eating invites a deeper connection to the food you eat and the world around you.

Chapter 16

Reducing Food Waste: Small Steps for Big Change

Food waste is becoming a bigger problem worldwide, with millions of tons of perfectly good food thrown away each year. The impact of this goes far beyond our kitchens—it wastes precious resources like water, energy, and labor, increases food insecurity, and harms the environment. When food ends up in landfills, it breaks down and releases methane, a harmful greenhouse gas that speeds up climate change.

The good news is that we don't need to make drastic changes to address this issue. Small, simple actions in our daily lives can make a big difference. Things like shopping smarter, storing food the right way, getting creative with leftovers, and composting can all help reduce waste.

In this chapter, we'll explore easy ways to cut down on food waste, from simple habits you can start in the kitchen to sustainable solutions like composting. We'll also discuss how being more mindful about the food we buy and eat can positively impact both our health and the planet. These small changes can help us save resources, cut down on waste, and build a more sustainable future for everyone.

Practical Tips for Reducing Food Waste in the Kitchen

The kitchen is not only the heart of the home but also the central stage for addressing one of the most pressing household challenges: food waste. It's where much of the unused, forgotten, or improperly stored food ends up in the trash. However, it's also where the greatest opportunities for meaningful change lie. Every decision made in the kitchen—from meal planning and food storage to cooking and composting—has the potential to reduce waste and foster a more sustainable lifestyle.

By adopting simple, actionable strategies, you can transform your kitchen into a space that reflects mindful consumption and resourcefulness. Reducing food waste isn't just about avoiding wastefulness; it's about creating a system where every ingredient is valued, utilized, and appreciated. These small but powerful changes not only help the environment by conserving resources and reducing landfill contributions but also bring practical benefits such as saving money, improving meal quality, and cultivating a sense of satisfaction in using food to its fullest potential.

With thoughtful planning and a shift in perspective, your kitchen can become a place where sustainability thrives and waste is minimized, setting a positive example for others in your household and beyond.

- **1. Plan Meals and Shop Smart**

Meal planning is a fundamental strategy for minimizing food waste, streamlining your grocery shopping, and optimizing your meals. By thoughtfully planning your weekly meals, you can ensure that every ingredient you purchase has a purpose, drastically reducing the likelihood of food going unused or forgotten in the back of the fridge. A well-structured meal plan allows you to align your shopping list with your actual needs, avoiding over-purchasing and helping you make the most of seasonal and perishable items.

Creating a detailed shopping list—and committing to it—is key to staying focused and avoiding the pitfalls of impulse buying. These unplanned purchases often lead to cluttered pantries and unused items, which ultimately contribute to waste. Meal planning also makes it easier to incorporate leftovers into future meals, ensuring that every bit of food is utilized. By adopting this practice, you can save money, reduce waste, and enjoy the peace of mind that comes with having a clear plan for your meals.

2. Proper Storage

Understanding how to store different foods can significantly extend their shelf life. For instance:

- Store leafy greens in a damp paper towel to keep them crisp.
- Keep fruits like bananas, apples, and avocados separate to prevent them from accelerating the ripening of other produce.
- Label and date leftovers to ensure they're eaten before they spoil.

3. Utilize Leftovers Creatively

Leftovers don't have to be boring. Transform last night's dinner into a new dish:

- Use roasted vegetables in a frittata or salad.
- Turn leftover rice into fried rice or a soup base.
- Blend overripe fruits into smoothies or freeze them for later use.

4. Embrace "Ugly" Produce

A staggering amount of perfectly edible fruits and vegetables are discarded before they even reach store shelves, solely because they don't meet strict aesthetic standards for size, shape, or color. These "imperfect" or "ugly" produce items may have minor blemishes or unconventional appearances, but they are just as nutritious and delicious as their picture-perfect counterparts. By choosing to purchase these underappreciated gems, you not only prevent unnecessary waste but also send a powerful message to producers and retailers about the value of all food.

Opting for imperfect produce often comes with the added benefit of cost savings, as these items are frequently sold at a lower price. Many grocery stores, farmers' markets, and specialty food delivery services now offer dedicated sections or boxes for "ugly" produce, making it easier than ever to embrace this sustainable choice. Supporting imperfect produce helps reduce the environmental burden of food waste, conserves resources used in production, and encourages a more inclusive food system where all produce, regardless of appearance, is valued.

5. Track and Adjust

Tracking your food waste is a simple yet powerful way to understand and address the habits contributing to it. Keeping a food waste diary for a week allows you to pinpoint recurring patterns, such as certain items that frequently go unused or portions that are consistently too large. Documenting what gets thrown away—noting the type of food, its condition, and the reason for disposal—can provide valuable insights into your shopping, cooking, and eating behaviors.

Once you've identified these patterns, you can take targeted steps to reduce waste. For instance, if you regularly discard wilted greens or spoiled dairy, consider buying smaller quantities or switching to shelf-stable alternatives. If leftovers often pile up uneaten, adjust portion sizes when cooking or incorporate those extras into your meal planning. This simple practice of reflection and adjustment can help you make more intentional choices, reduce food waste, and create a more efficient and sustainable kitchen routine.

Composting: Turning Scraps into Valuable Resources

When food scraps do occur, composting offers an effective way to recycle them into nutrient-rich soil. This process not only reduces waste but also contributes to healthier gardens and less reliance on chemical fertilizers.

1. What Can Be Composted?

Most food scraps can be composted, including:

- Fruit and vegetable peels
- Coffee grounds and tea bags
- Eggshells
- Bread and grains (in moderation)

However, avoid composting meat, dairy, and oily foods, as these can attract pests and slow the composting process.

2. Setting Up a Compost System

Composting can be done in various ways depending on your space and resources:

- **Backyard Composting:** Ideal for those with outdoor space, this involves creating a compost pile or using a bin.
- **Indoor Composting:** Compact compost bins with carbon filters are perfect for apartments.
- **Community Composting:** Many urban areas offer community composting programs where residents can drop off food scraps.

3. The Benefits of Composting

Composting not only diverts food waste from landfills but also enriches soil, improving its ability to retain water and nutrients. Using compost in your garden reduces the need for chemical fertilizers and supports healthier plants.

Mindful Consumption: A Shift in Perspective

Mindful consumption is a holistic approach to food that emphasizes intentionality, awareness, and responsibility in our daily choices. It goes beyond simply buying and eating food—it's about cultivating a deeper connection to what we consume and understanding the broader implications of those decisions. This practice encourages us to reflect on the journey of our food, from how it's grown and transported to how it's prepared and ultimately disposed of.

At its core, mindful consumption invites us to buy only what we need, prioritize quality over quantity, and choose sustainably produced and locally sourced foods whenever possible. It means being attentive to portion sizes, embracing leftovers, and finding creative ways to use every part of an ingredient to minimize waste. Preparing meals thoughtfully and savoring them fully also fosters a greater appreciation for the resources and effort that go into every bite.

Moreover, mindful consumption promotes sustainable habits by reducing over-purchasing, supporting ethical food systems, and contributing to a healthier planet. It empowers us to make choices that align with our values, whether that's reducing our carbon footprint, supporting local farmers, or simply wasting less. Ultimately, mindful consumption is not just a way to eat but a way to live—with gratitude, awareness, and a commitment to sustainability.

1. Buy What You Need

Over-purchasing is a major contributor to food waste. Be realistic about the amount of food your household can consume and resist buying in bulk unless you're sure it will be used.

2. Respect Expiration Dates

Understanding food labels can prevent unnecessary waste:

- **"Best Before" Dates:** Indicate peak quality, not safety. Many foods are still edible after this date.
- **"Use By" Dates:** Should be adhered to for safety reasons, particularly with perishable items.

3. Eat Smaller Portions

Serving smaller portions reduces the likelihood of uneaten food. Seconds are always an option if someone is still hungry.

4. Support Food Recovery Programs

If you have surplus food, consider donating to local food banks or recovery programs that redistribute edible food to those in need.

5. Educate and Involve Others

Encourage friends and family to adopt waste-reducing practices. Share tips, recipes, and the benefits of sustainable living to create a ripple effect of positive change.

The Bigger Picture: Environmental and Economic Impact

Reducing food waste isn't just about saving scraps—it's about acknowledging the resources and energy that go into food production. Every discarded apple or loaf of bread represents water, land, labor, and transportation resources that are ultimately wasted. By reducing food waste, we contribute to:

- Lower greenhouse gas emissions
- Reduced strain on landfills
- Conservation of water and energy resources
- Alleviation of global food insecurity

Reducing food waste is a simple yet profoundly impactful step toward building a more sustainable future. Small, intentional actions in the kitchen—such as smarter meal planning, proper food storage, and creative use of leftovers—can significantly reduce the amount of food we waste. Embracing composting further amplifies this effort by turning unavoidable scraps into valuable resources that enrich the soil and support healthier ecosystems.

Adopting mindful consumption habits encourages us to value food as the precious resource it is, fostering a deeper awareness of the effort and resources required to bring it to our plates. These changes not only save money and improve personal health but also play a critical role in addressing environmental challenges like climate change, resource depletion, and landfill overflows. By transforming wasteful behaviors into sustainable practices, we contribute to a healthier planet and set a positive example for future generations, demonstrating that even small actions can lead to meaningful, long-lasting change.

Chapter 17

The Psychology of Healthy Eating

Eating is far more than just a physical necessity—it's a deeply ingrained part of our daily lives, influenced by emotions, behaviors, and even cultural norms. What we choose to eat and how we feel about food are shaped by a wide array of psychological factors. These influences can impact our eating habits in both positive and negative ways, making it essential to explore the psychology behind food choices if we want to build lasting, healthy habits. Understanding how emotions, stress, and even environmental cues trigger food cravings and emotional eating can help us gain more control over our eating behaviors.

This chapter will explore these psychological forces, focusing on the impact of food cravings and emotional eating, and provide actionable insights into how we can combat these tendencies. We'll look at how food marketing, societal pressures, and personal beliefs can influence what we eat, and we'll offer strategies for becoming more aware of these external influences.

In addition, we'll delve into how to build sustainable, healthy habits that go beyond temporary dietary changes. Instead of focusing on restrictive diets or quick fixes, we'll explore how to create a lasting shift in mindset and behavior that supports overall well-being. Healthy eating isn't just about the food we choose; it's about developing a healthy relationship with food and learning to listen to our bodies.

The chapter will also provide practical advice on staying committed to your sustainable eating goals. For many of us, staying on track can be the hardest part, especially when faced with challenges like stress, cravings, or societal pressures to eat in ways that don't align with our values. We'll offer strategies to help you stay motivated and focused on your goals, making it easier to incorporate healthier, sustainable eating into your everyday life.

By the end of this chapter, you'll have a deeper understanding of the psychological aspects that influence your eating habits, along with the tools to build healthier, more sustainable relationships with food. These insights will empower you to take control of your food choices, reduce emotional eating, and establish habits that will help you maintain a balanced, sustainable diet for life.

Understanding Food Cravings and Emotional Eating

Food cravings are a powerful force. They can hit us suddenly, leaving us feeling almost powerless against the urge to indulge. While cravings can sometimes be physical—such as when our bodies need a specific nutrient—many cravings are driven by psychological and emotional factors. Understanding the root causes of these cravings is the first step in overcoming them and creating healthier eating habits.

The Science of Food Cravings

Food cravings are often linked to changes in our brain chemistry. When we eat foods high in sugar, fat, or salt, our brains release dopamine, the "feel-good" chemical. This creates a sense of pleasure and satisfaction, which can reinforce our desire to eat those foods again. This cycle of reward can become addictive, making it hard to resist cravings, especially when we're stressed, bored, or feeling down.

However, it's not just the food itself that triggers cravings—it's also the way our brains associate certain foods with specific feelings or situations. For example, we may crave comfort foods when we're feeling stressed, lonely, or sad, because our brains associate those foods with emotional relief.

Emotional Eating: A Coping Mechanism

Emotional eating is a coping mechanism that many of us use to deal with difficult emotions or stress. When we experience negative feelings such as anxiety, depression, or frustration, food can provide a temporary distraction or a sense of comfort. This can lead to overeating, eating unhealthy foods, or using food to numb emotions, rather than nourish our bodies.

The problem with emotional eating is that it doesn't address the underlying emotions. While food may provide a temporary sense of relief, it doesn't solve the emotional issue at hand. In fact, it can often make us feel worse, especially if we overeat and then feel guilty or ashamed. Over time, emotional eating can create a pattern of unhealthy habits, making it more difficult to maintain a balanced diet and make conscious food choices.

Breaking the Cycle of Cravings and Emotional Eating

The key to overcoming cravings and emotional eating lies in developing healthier coping mechanisms and increasing self-awareness. Here are a few strategies that can help:

- **Mindful Eating** : Practicing mindfulness during meals allows us to slow down, pay attention to our food, and recognize when we're full. This practice can help us differentiate between physical hunger and emotional cravings. When we eat mindfully, we're more likely to make conscious, intentional food choices, which can reduce the likelihood of overeating or reaching for unhealthy comfort foods.

- **Stress Management** : Emotional eating often occurs as a response to stress, so it's important to find healthier ways to cope with stress. Practices such as yoga, meditation, deep breathing, and regular physical activity can help reduce stress levels and prevent emotional eating triggers.
- **Emotional Awareness** : Learning to identify and address the emotions that lead to emotional eating is essential. Keeping an emotional food journal can help you track patterns and recognize when you tend to eat in response to specific feelings. Once you're aware of these triggers, you can take proactive steps to address the root cause of your emotions, rather than turning to food for comfort.
- **Seek Support** : Sometimes, it's helpful to talk to a therapist or counselor about your relationship with food. They can help you explore the emotional factors contributing to emotional eating and work with you on strategies to develop healthier coping mechanisms.

How to Build Healthy, Lasting Habits

Building healthy eating habits takes time, patience, and commitment. It's not about making drastic changes overnight, but rather about making gradual improvements that are sustainable in the long term. To build lasting habits, it's important to focus on consistency, self-compassion, and positive reinforcement.

1. Start Small and Set Achievable Goals

Trying to make too many changes at once can be overwhelming. Instead, start small and set realistic, achievable goals. For example, if you want to eat more vegetables, begin by adding one extra serving to your meals each day, rather than committing to a complete diet overhaul. Gradually increase the number of healthy foods in your diet as you become more comfortable with these changes.

Setting specific, measurable goals is important for tracking progress and staying motivated. Whether it's cooking at home three nights a week or swapping sugary snacks for healthier options, small, incremental changes are more sustainable than trying to do everything at once.

2. Create a Supportive Environment

Your environment plays a big role in shaping your eating habits. Surround yourself with healthy food options and remove tempting, unhealthy foods from your home. Stock your kitchen with fresh fruits, vegetables, whole grains, and lean proteins, and plan your meals ahead of time to ensure you have the ingredients you need for nutritious meals. By setting yourself up for success, you make it easier to stick to your goals.

It can also be helpful to share your goals with others. Having a support system can provide encouragement and accountability, making it easier to stay committed to your healthy eating goals. Whether it's a friend, family member, or a community group, finding people who share your values can help you stay motivated and inspired.

3. Practice Self-Compassion

Building healthy habits is a journey, and it's normal to encounter setbacks along the way. It's important to be kind to yourself during this process. If you slip up and eat something unhealthy, don't beat yourself up. Instead, view it as a learning opportunity and move forward with a positive mindset. Self-compassion helps reduce feelings of guilt and shame, which can often lead to emotional eating and negative cycles.

4. Celebrate Progress

Celebrating small victories along the way is essential for building lasting habits. Whether it's acknowledging a week of successful meal prep or recognizing the fact that you've reduced your intake of processed foods, take the time to celebrate your progress. Positive reinforcement helps build confidence and motivates you to continue your healthy eating journey.

Staying Committed to Your Sustainable Eating Goals

Once you've set your goals and started building healthy habits, the next challenge is staying committed to your sustainable eating goals. There will be times when you're tempted to stray from your plan, whether due to stress, busy schedules, or social pressures. The key is to stay focused, stay flexible, and remember why you started in the first place.

1. Plan Ahead

Meal planning is one of the best ways to stay on track with your sustainable eating goals. By planning your meals in advance, you ensure that you always have nutritious options available and reduce the temptation to resort to convenience foods. You can plan meals that are easy to prepare, use up leftovers, and incorporate a variety of healthy ingredients to keep things interesting.

2. Learn to Navigate Social Situations

Social events, dining out, and celebrations can pose challenges to maintaining your healthy eating goals. However, with a little planning and flexibility, you can navigate these situations without feeling deprived. Eat a healthy snack before heading out, so you're not overly hungry when you arrive at a party, and always feel free to politely decline foods that don't align with your goals. Most importantly, remember that one indulgence doesn't ruin your progress—it's the overall consistency that counts.

3. Track Your Progress

Tracking your food choices, progress, and emotional triggers can help you stay connected to your goals and keep you accountable. Use a food journal or an app to log your meals, emotions, and any challenges you encounter. This will give you insight into areas where you're succeeding and areas that might need more attention.

4. Be Flexible

Sometimes life throws us curve balls, and sticking to a rigid eating plan isn't always possible. That's okay. It's important to be flexible and adapt your plan when necessary. Whether it's adjusting your meal prep for a busy week or allowing yourself an occasional treat, flexibility ensures that your sustainable eating goals remain achievable over the long term.

The psychology of healthy eating is far more intricate than simply knowing what foods are good for us. It's deeply intertwined with our emotions, behaviors, and environment, all of which shape our food choices and eating patterns. By gaining a deeper understanding of the psychological factors that drive food cravings and emotional eating, we can begin to make conscious, intentional decisions that break free from unhealthy cycles and help us build lasting, positive habits.

Building healthy eating habits isn't an overnight process; it requires patience, self-awareness, and a strong commitment to change. It's about shifting our mindset and developing a more mindful approach to food, one that is rooted in self-care rather than restriction. By embracing mindful eating, setting small, achievable goals, and acknowledging the progress we make along the way, we can steadily work towards a more sustainable and balanced way of eating.

The road to healthier eating is a journey, but with the right strategies and mindset, we can create lasting change. We can learn to listen to our bodies, make more intentional food choices, and stay committed to our goals, even in the face of challenges. Ultimately, these steps not only help us achieve our sustainable eating goals but also lead to a healthier, more balanced life that nourishes both our bodies and minds.

Chapter 18

Mindful Eating: Reconnecting with Food

In our days, living in fast-paced world, where food is often seen as nothing more than fuel, something to be consumed quickly to check off another task on our never-ending to-do lists. Whether we're eating in the car, snacking at our desks, or scrolling through our phones while eating dinner, we've become disconnected from the true essence of food. We're no longer fully present during meals, often eating mindlessly or distractedly, which can lead to poor digestion, overeating, and a loss of appreciation for the nourishment food provides. The growing rate of processed foods, eating on the go, and multitasking during meals has distanced us from the joy and purpose that food once held in our lives.

Enter mindful eating—a practice that offers us a way to reconnect with food and embrace a more thoughtful, conscious approach to eating. Rooted in ancient practices like mindfulness meditation, mindful eating encourages us to slow down, pay attention to the present moment, and truly engage with the act of eating. It's about being present with your food—observing its colors, textures, and smells, appreciating each bite, and listening to your body's signals of hunger and fullness. Mindful eating isn't just about what you eat; it's about how you eat. It's an approach that can help improve digestion, foster healthier relationships with food, and reduce overeating by encouraging us to savor our meals rather than rush through them.

At the heart of mindful eating is the idea of cultivating awareness and presence during mealtime. It's about slowing down, savoring the flavors, and reconnecting with the act of eating in a way that nurtures our bodies and minds. This chapter will guide you through the concept of mindful eating, explore its numerous health benefits, and provide practical tips for how to incorporate mindfulness into your everyday meals. We'll delve into how practicing mindful eating can not only improve your overall health but also help reduce overeating and prevent the mindless consumption that has become so common in modern life.

When we practice mindful eating, we bring our full attention to the food in front of us. We notice the vibrant colors of vegetables, the texture of grains, the warmth of a freshly baked dish. By focusing on these sensory aspects, we create a deeper connection with our food. Eating mindfully allows us to truly savor and appreciate the flavors, making every bite more fulfilling and satisfying. This practice can also help us eat more slowly, giving our bodies time to process hunger and fullness cues, which is crucial for preventing overeating and making healthier choices.

Mindful eating also helps us rebuild our intuition around food. In a world where we are constantly bombarded with diet trends and food rules, it can be easy to lose touch with what our bodies truly need. Mindful eating encourages us to listen to our bodies rather than external cues—like a calorie count or social pressure—to determine when and how much to eat. By tuning into our hunger signals and eating only until we are comfortably full, we can avoid the discomfort and guilt that often comes with overeating.

Moreover, mindful eating can help us develop a healthier relationship with food by reducing emotional eating. When we eat mindfully, we're better able to distinguish between true physical hunger and emotional triggers, such as stress or boredom. Mindful eating encourages us to slow down and create space between emotional responses and eating, allowing us to make more intentional choices about how we nourish ourselves.

As we explore the concept of mindful eating in this chapter, we will not only focus on how to eat more mindfully, but also on the broader benefits that mindful eating can bring to our overall well-being. From improving digestion to fostering a sense of gratitude and enjoyment, mindful eating offers a holistic approach to food that goes beyond what's on our plate. This practice can help us reconnect with the deep nourishment food provides, promote better digestion and absorption of nutrients, and cultivate a more positive, sustainable approach to eating.

We will provide practical guidance on how to implement mindful eating into your daily routine, offering actionable steps to integrate mindfulness into mealtime. You'll learn simple techniques like chewing slowly, pausing between bites, and taking a few deep breaths before eating. We'll also discuss how you can be more intentional in choosing foods that support your health, the environment, and your ethical values. Whether you're sitting down for a quiet dinner or grabbing a snack on the go, these tips will help you cultivate awareness and mindfulness in every meal.

Ultimately, this chapter aims to guide you toward a more conscious, balanced, and satisfying relationship with food. By practicing mindful eating, we can transform our approach to meals, reduce overeating, and truly savor the experience of eating. Through small but powerful changes in the way we eat, we can nourish both our bodies and our minds, contributing to a healthier, more sustainable, and more fulfilling life. Mindful eating is not just a diet or a trend—it's a way of living that encourages us to embrace food with intention, gratitude, and presence.

As we embark on this journey of mindful eating, let's remember that food is more than just something to fill our stomachs—it's an opportunity to nourish ourselves holistically, from the inside out. By eating mindfully, we are reclaiming our relationship with food, fostering a deeper appreciation for the meals we consume, and making choices that support both our health and the planet.

What Is Mindful Eating and How Does It Promote Health?

Mindful eating is rooted in the practice of mindfulness—a concept derived from Buddhist teachings that involves being fully present and aware in the moment, without judgment. In the context of eating, mindfulness means paying full attention to the experience of eating, from the sight and smell of food to the taste, texture, and sensations of each bite. It involves engaging all your senses, noticing how the food makes you feel, and tuning into your hunger and fullness cues.

When we eat mindfully, we shift away from mindless habits like eating while watching TV or rushing through meals. Instead, we approach food with curiosity and gratitude, acknowledging the nourishment it provides. This practice not only enhances the pleasure and satisfaction we derive from eating but also supports our physical and emotional well-being.

One of the core principles of mindful eating is the awareness of how our body feels before, during, and after a meal. Research has shown that this awareness can significantly improve digestion, promote healthier eating patterns, and even lead to weight loss. Studies indicate that when we eat mindfully, we are more likely to make healthier food choices, eat in appropriate portions, and feel more satisfied with our meals. It allows us to respond to our body's hunger signals and avoid overeating or emotional eating.

Mindful eating also helps reduce the stress and anxiety that often surround food. Many people experience guilt or shame after overeating, or they may engage in restrictive diets, creating a negative cycle around food. Mindful eating encourages self-compassion and a more balanced approach to nourishment. By letting go of the food rules and labels that can be mentally exhausting, we can foster a healthier, more positive relationship with food.

Practicing Mindfulness at Mealtime

The process of practicing mindful eating can be broken down into several simple steps, each designed to help you focus more deeply on the experience of eating and the food itself. Incorporating mindfulness into mealtimes can transform your eating habits, improve digestion, and help you enjoy food on a deeper level.

1. Set the Scene:
To begin, create a calm and distraction-free environment for your meals. This means turning off the TV, putting away your phone, and sitting down at a table where you can focus on the food in front of you. This simple step allows you to fully engage in the experience without being distracted by external stimuli. You may want to create a peaceful atmosphere by lighting a candle, playing soothing music, or practicing deep breathing before you begin your meal.

2. Observe the Food:
Before taking the first bite, take a moment to simply look at your food. Notice the colors, textures, and arrangement of the meal. Appreciate the effort that went into preparing the food and the nourishment it will provide. Observe the food as if you were seeing it for the first time. This step helps you connect with the food in a meaningful way and cultivates gratitude for the meal.

3. Engage Your Senses:
As you begin eating, use all your senses to fully experience the food. Notice the aroma, the taste, the temperature, and the texture. Try to focus on each bite and savor the flavors as they unfold. Take smaller bites and chew slowly, paying attention to how the food feels in your mouth. The more you engage your senses, the more enjoyable and satisfying the meal will be.

4. Tune Into Hunger and Fullness Cues:
Mindful eating also involves paying attention to your body's internal signals of hunger and fullness. Before eating, ask yourself if you're truly hungry or if you're eating out of boredom, stress, or habit. During the meal, check in with yourself periodically to gauge how full you feel. It can be helpful to pause midway through your meal to assess your level of satisfaction. Eating slowly and mindfully allows your body to signal when it's had enough, preventing overeating and promoting more balanced portions.

5. Reflect on the Meal:
Once you've finished eating, take a moment to reflect on how the meal made you feel. Are you satisfied and energized, or do you feel sluggish or overfull? Notice the physical sensations in your body, and check in with your emotions. Reflecting on your meal can help you understand your body's needs better and learn from the experience, whether it was enjoyable or less satisfying.

How to Savor Food and Reduce Overeating

Mindful eating can be particularly helpful in combating overeating. In a world where portion sizes are often oversized and eating habits are rushed, it's easy to consume more food than we need. Mindfulness encourages us to listen to our body's cues and honor our hunger and fullness, leading to more balanced eating habits.

Savoring the Food:
Savoring food is an important aspect of mindful eating. Savoring means taking the time to truly enjoy and appreciate the flavors and textures of the food you're eating. When we savor our meals, we tend to feel more satisfied, even with smaller portions. This is because we are focused on the enjoyment of the food, rather than simply eating to finish a meal quickly or out of habit.

Research shows that when we savor food, we become more aware of how much we're eating, which helps reduce the likelihood of overeating. Savoring also enhances the pleasure we get from food, allowing us to feel more satisfied and content without needing to eat large amounts.

Slow Down and Eat with Intention:
Slowing down is a key element of mindful eating that can help reduce overeating. When we eat too quickly, we often don't give our brains enough time to register that we're full. By eating more slowly, we give our body the time it needs to send signals to our brain that it's had enough, helping to prevent overeating. Aim to chew each bite thoroughly and pause between bites to give yourself the opportunity to assess how full you feel.

Mindful eating also encourages eating with intention. This means being conscious of what you're eating and why you're eating it. It may be helpful to ask yourself whether you're eating because you're truly hungry, or if you're eating for other reasons, such as stress, boredom, or social pressure. Being intentional about eating can help break the cycle of emotional or mindless eating and promote more balanced food choices.

Portion Control and Moderation:
Mindful eating encourages portion control in a natural and intuitive way. By paying attention to your hunger and fullness cues, you can learn to eat the right amount of food for your body. This approach fosters a healthy relationship with food, without the need for restrictive diets or calorie counting. Mindful eating teaches moderation and helps you avoid overeating, as you become more in tune with your body's needs.

Reconnecting with Food for a Healthier Life

Mindful eating is not just a technique—it's a powerful, transformative approach that has the potential to reshape both our health and our relationship with food. In a world where eating is often rushed or distracted, practicing mindfulness at mealtime allows us to slow down, truly savor what we're eating, and become more in tune with our body's natural cues. By paying attention to the textures, flavors, and aromas of our food, we cultivate a deeper connection to the nourishment it provides. This practice empowers us to make healthier food choices, reduces the likelihood of overeating, and alleviates the guilt and stress that frequently accompany our food-related decisions.

Through mindful eating, we rediscover the simple pleasure of eating—something that many of us have lost touch with in our busy, fast-paced lives. It encourages us to eat with intention, promoting a healthier relationship with food and our bodies. As we slow down and approach food with gratitude, we not only improve our digestion and satisfaction but also make room for more sustainable and conscious food habits. This process encourages us to focus on what our bodies truly need, instead of simply responding to external cues like portion sizes or emotional triggers.

Furthermore, mindful eating nurtures a more balanced, nourishing lifestyle. By embracing this approach, we can create positive patterns that benefit both our physical health and our emotional well-being. It also has the potential to impact the environment by encouraging us to make food choices that are more sustainable and aligned with our values. When we approach food with mindfulness, we become more aware of the resources that go into producing it and develop a greater sense of responsibility toward what we consume.

By practicing mindful eating, we can transform our relationship with food, foster a healthier mindset, and contribute to a more harmonious connection with both our bodies and the planet. Each mindful meal is an opportunity to nourish ourselves holistically—body, mind, and spirit—promoting well-being and sustainability in one conscious act of eating.

Chapter 19

The Role of Hydration in Your Diet

Water is not just a beverage; it's the lifeblood of our bodies. It is a critical component of every cell, tissue, and organ, making it essential for maintaining all aspects of physical health. Water plays a central role in virtually every bodily function, from the absorption and transportation of nutrients to the regulation of body temperature and the removal of waste. Every single process within our body, from metabolism to immune function, relies on hydration. Despite the overwhelming evidence of water's significance, many people still neglect hydration, focusing more on food or exercise and overlooking this foundational aspect of health.

When you think about it, hydration is involved in everything your body does. It helps break down food during digestion, allowing nutrients to be absorbed effectively. It regulates body temperature by carrying heat away from your organs and tissues. Water also acts as a lubricant for your joints, preventing friction and promoting smooth movement. On top of that, it's essential for delivering oxygen to cells and aiding in the body's detoxification processes. Without enough water, these functions slow down, which can lead to fatigue, poor concentration, digestive issues, and a variety of other health concerns.

The importance of water extends far beyond just quenching thirst. While thirst is the body's natural signal for hydration, by the time we feel thirsty, our bodies may already be in a mild state of dehydration. Chronic dehydration can lead to a range of problems, from headaches and dry skin to more serious conditions like kidney stones, urinary tract infections, and even cognitive decline. It's essential to stay ahead of our body's needs and keep hydration levels up throughout the day.

But proper hydration isn't just a matter of drinking water—it's about incorporating water-rich foods into our diets, listening to our bodies, and finding sustainable solutions to ensure we stay hydrated. Many people rely heavily on bottled water, often unaware of the environmental costs involved. Bottled water requires vast amounts of plastic production, transportation, and energy consumption. Not to mention, a significant amount of plastic waste ends up in landfills and oceans, contributing to pollution and climate change. The good news is, there are plenty of sustainable alternatives that can help reduce our ecological footprint without compromising on hydration. Reusable water bottles, home filtration systems, and even the habit of filling up at water refill stations or using eco-friendly filtration options can significantly reduce the demand for bottled water and help protect the planet.

In this chapter, we will also explore how to make hydration a part of your daily routine in a way that is sustainable for both you and the environment. We will discuss strategies for drinking more water throughout the day, how to identify your body's unique hydration needs, and how to gauge if you're drinking enough. Additionally, we will address hydration myths and provide tips for ensuring that your body is getting the water it needs. When we approach hydration with intention and mindfulness, we can support our body's systems while making choices that are also beneficial for the planet's future.

The Importance of Water for Overall Health

Water makes up about 60% of the human body, and it's crucial to nearly every function. It acts as a solvent, dissolving nutrients, minerals, and compounds so that the body can absorb them. It also helps regulate body temperature through sweating and respiration, cushions joints, and eliminates waste products through urine. Without water, our bodies wouldn't be able to function optimally, and our health would deteriorate rapidly.

One of water's most essential roles is in digestion. It helps break down food so that your body can absorb the nutrients it needs. Additionally, water assists in the transportation of these nutrients to cells throughout the body via the bloodstream. Without sufficient hydration, the digestion process becomes less efficient, leading to issues like constipation or bloating.

Water also plays a crucial role in maintaining the balance of bodily fluids, including electrolytes like sodium, potassium, and calcium. These are vital for muscle function, nerve signaling, and maintaining normal heart rhythms. Dehydration can disrupt this delicate balance, leading to fatigue, muscle cramps, headaches, and other serious conditions.

The brain is another major beneficiary of water. Staying hydrated enhances cognitive function, improves concentration, and boosts memory. Dehydration, on the other hand, can impair mood, reduce focus, and increase stress levels. This is why even mild dehydration can lead to feelings of sluggishness, irritability, and difficulty concentrating.

The Dangers of Dehydration

Dehydration can have serious, immediate effects on the body, especially when it's left unaddressed. Mild dehydration can cause fatigue, headaches, and dizziness, while severe dehydration can lead to confusion, organ failure, and even death. The symptoms of dehydration often include a dry mouth, dark urine, a decrease in urine output, and a feeling of extreme thirst.

One of the challenges in maintaining proper hydration is that the body's signals for thirst can be easily overlooked or ignored. By the time we feel thirsty, we are already mildly dehydrated. Many of us confuse thirst with hunger, leading to unnecessary snacking when our bodies actually need water. As a result, we may not realize that dehydration can contribute to overeating or unhealthy food choices.

In addition to the immediate effects, chronic dehydration can contribute to the development of various health problems. These include kidney stones, urinary tract infections, bladder infections, and even chronic constipation. Furthermore, studies have shown that prolonged dehydration can affect skin health, leading to dryness and the formation of wrinkles over time.

Sustainable Alternatives to Bottled Water

Bottled water is one of the most widely consumed beverages globally. While it's convenient, it comes with significant environmental costs. The production of plastic bottles contributes to pollution, with millions of bottles ending up in landfills or oceans each year. In fact, it's estimated that around 1 million plastic bottles are sold every minute, and the vast majority of these bottles are not recycled. This waste contributes to the growing issue of plastic pollution, which harms wildlife and ecosystems.

In addition to the environmental impact, bottled water is often much more expensive than tap water, even though the quality is frequently similar. In many countries, tap water is subject to strict regulations and is often just as clean and safe to drink as bottled water. By switching from bottled water to sustainable alternatives, we can help reduce plastic waste and contribute to a more eco-friendly lifestyle.

Here are a few sustainable alternatives to bottled water:

- **Reusable Water Bottles:** Investing in a high-quality, reusable water bottle is one of the easiest and most effective ways to reduce plastic waste. With a variety of sizes, designs, and materials available (including stainless steel, glass, and BPA-free plastic), reusable bottles are both convenient and eco-friendly. You can carry your bottle with you throughout the day and refill it as needed.

- **Water Filtration Systems:** For those who are concerned about the quality of their tap water, investing in a water filtration system can be a great option. There are many different types of filters available, ranging from simple pitcher filters to more advanced under-sink filtration systems. These filters can help remove contaminants like chlorine, lead, and other impurities, making tap water taste better and safer to drink.

- **Water Refill Stations:** Many public places, including gyms, schools, and airports, are increasingly offering water refill stations where you can fill your reusable bottle. These stations help reduce reliance on bottled water and provide a convenient way to stay hydrated while out and about.

- **Water from Natural Sources:** If you live in an area with access to clean natural water sources, such as spring water, you may be able to collect your own water. Just make sure that the water has been tested for safety and that the collection process doesn't harm the environment.

How to Ensure You're Drinking Enough Water Each Day

While the amount of water each person needs can vary significantly depending on factors like age, sex, physical activity levels, and the climate in which they live, there are general guidelines that can help ensure proper hydration. One popular recommendation is the "8x8 rule," which suggests drinking eight 8-ounce glasses of water a day. While this is a straightforward and easy-to-remember guideline, hydration needs are not one-size-fits-all. Experts suggest that a more personalized approach might be necessary, as individual factors play a significant role in how much water we require.

For example, people who are more physically active may need more water to replace the fluids lost through sweat, while those living in hot or humid climates may also require higher amounts of hydration to combat the effects of heat. Additionally, certain health conditions, like kidney issues or pregnancy, can affect hydration needs, making it important to listen to your body and adjust accordingly.

Moreover, hydration isn't just about drinking water—it's about getting fluids from various sources, including fruits, vegetables, and other beverages. Foods like cucumbers, watermelon, and oranges are rich in water and can complement your daily hydration intake. So, while the "8x8" rule serves as a good starting point, staying in tune with your body's cues and considering the factors that influence your water needs will ensure you're properly hydrated throughout the day.

Signs You May Need More Water:

- Dark-colored urine: If your urine is dark yellow or amber, it may indicate dehydration. Clear or light yellow urine is generally a sign of proper hydration.
- Dry mouth and lips: If you feel your mouth or lips getting dry throughout the day, it could be a sign that you need more fluids.
- Fatigue: Dehydration can cause feelings of fatigue and sluggishness, as your body works harder to maintain its functions.
- Headaches: Mild dehydration can trigger headaches or migraines, which may worsen if you don't rehydrate.
- Dizziness or confusion: In more severe cases of dehydration, you may experience dizziness, lightheadedness, or confusion.

Tips to Stay Hydrated:

- **Drink Water Consistently:** Rather than waiting until you're thirsty, try to sip water throughout the day. Keep a water bottle handy and take regular, small sips to maintain hydration levels.
- **Eat Hydrating Foods:** Many fruits and vegetables, such as watermelon, cucumbers, and oranges, contain high amounts of water and can contribute to hydration. Incorporating these foods into your diet can help you stay hydrated.
- **Track Your Intake:** Use a hydration app or set reminders on your phone to help you remember to drink water at regular intervals.
- **Hydrate Before, During, and After Exercise:** If you're physically active, it's important to drink water

before, during, and after your workout to replace fluids lost through sweat.
- **Set Hydration Goals:** Setting a daily hydration goal, such as aiming for a specific number of glasses of water, can help keep you on track.

Water is truly the foundation of life, playing an integral role in maintaining our overall well-being. Staying properly hydrated goes far beyond just quenching thirst —it is essential for every function of our bodies. Hydration impacts everything from digestion and nutrient absorption to energy levels, cognitive performance, and emotional balance. Whether you're feeling sluggish, struggling with focus, or experiencing headaches, dehydration might be the hidden cause. Making hydration a priority in your daily routine has profound benefits, not just for your body but also for your mind and mood.

In today's world, it's also essential to consider the environmental impact of how we hydrate. The over-reliance on bottled water contributes to plastic waste and environmental degradation, further stressing the importance of switching to more sustainable alternatives like reusable bottles, water filtration systems, or using public water refill stations. By shifting towards these greener options, we can help reduce the plastic waste crisis while ensuring we remain properly hydrated.

It's also important to remember that hydration is not a one-size-fits-all process—our water needs can vary based on activity levels, climate, and individual factors. Developing habits like drinking consistently throughout the day, incorporating hydrating foods into your diet, and tuning in to your body's signals for thirst are simple but effective ways to keep hydration at optimal levels. The key lies in creating a balance between drinking enough water and making conscious choices that benefit both our health and the planet.

When we take the time to understand the critical role hydration plays in our lives and commit to ensuring we're drinking enough water, we're not only investing in our physical health and energy but also in a more sustainable and conscientious future. With every sip, we're making choices that nurture our bodies, support our environment, and help create a lasting, positive impact on the world.

Chapter 20

Supplements: Do You Need Them?

Supplements have become a key element in the pursuit of optimal health in today's society. With so much information and a wide variety of options on the market, it can be overwhelming to navigate the supplement landscape. From multivitamins to specialized formulas, the sheer volume of choices can leave us wondering: Do we really need them? When should we consider using supplements, and how do we incorporate them in a way that doesn't overshadow the nutritional value of whole foods?

The reality is that while supplements can indeed offer valuable support in filling nutritional gaps and addressing specific health needs, they are not a replacement for a balanced, nutrient-rich diet. Whole foods—fruits, vegetables, whole grains, legumes, nuts, seeds, and lean proteins—should always form the foundation of a healthy lifestyle. These foods are packed with the essential nutrients our bodies need to function at their best. However, in today's fast-paced world where diets may be restricted for various reasons or where soil depletion has reduced the nutrient density of our food, supplements can help fill the gaps.

The key to using supplements wisely lies in understanding when they are truly necessary. This involves identifying specific deficiencies or health concerns that can be addressed with targeted supplementation, such as vitamin D for those with limited sun exposure or omega-3 fatty acids for those not consuming enough fatty fish. When used properly, supplements can support overall health and well-being, helping you thrive. However, it's essential to choose supplements that are aligned with your personal health goals and sourced from ethical, sustainable, and natural methods. This is especially important as many synthetic supplements can contain additives, fillers, and questionable ingredients that can do more harm than good in the long run.

Sustainable and natural supplements are growing in popularity, as more consumers seek products that align with their values. Plant-based and organic supplements offer a cleaner, more environmentally friendly option, often free from harmful chemicals and pesticides. Choosing supplements that are responsibly sourced, cruelty-free, and eco-conscious can enhance the positive impact you're already making with your food choices. Whether it's a plant-based vitamin B12 supplement or a sustainably harvested fish oil, the sourcing and environmental impact of your supplement choices are just as important as their intended health benefits.

Incorporating supplements into a balanced diet requires a mindful approach, ensuring that they enhance—not replace—the nutrition you are getting from whole foods. Rather than relying on supplements as a quick fix, think of them as an addition to a strong dietary foundation. The goal should always be to prioritize whole, fresh foods first and turn to supplements when specific needs arise.

Ultimately, achieving optimal health isn't just about the supplements we take—it's about the overall lifestyle choices we make, from the foods we eat to the ways we live. By integrating mindful, intentional supplementation with a focus on nourishing, sustainable foods, we can achieve a balanced, holistic approach to health. This chapter will guide you through the process of assessing when supplements are necessary, selecting the best natural options, and ensuring they complement your diet for the most effective, health-supporting results. Together, we can create a health plan that nourishes our bodies and respects the planet, helping us thrive in every aspect of life.

When and Why to Consider Supplements

Most people are familiar with the general concept of supplements—pills or powders that supposedly boost our health by filling gaps in our diet. In some cases, they can help ensure we're getting enough essential nutrients that might be lacking in our food. But while many supplements are widely available, it's crucial to consider when and why you might need them.

1. Nutrient Deficiencies

The primary reason for taking supplements is to address nutrient deficiencies. While a balanced diet should ideally provide all the essential vitamins, minerals, and other nutrients we need, modern lifestyles, food production methods, and environmental factors can lead to gaps in our nutrition. For example, certain individuals might need additional nutrients due to specific conditions such as pregnancy, age, health problems, or dietary restrictions.

Common deficiencies include:

- **Vitamin D** : Many people, particularly those living in colder climates or who don't get regular sun exposure, are deficient in vitamin D. This vitamin is crucial for bone health, immune function, and mood regulation.

- **Iron** : Women of childbearing age or people with a vegan or vegetarian diet may be at risk for iron deficiency, which can lead to anemia and fatigue.
- **Vitamin B12** : This vitamin is primarily found in animal products, so vegetarians and vegans might not get enough of it, leading to fatigue, memory problems, and nerve damage if left unaddressed.

In these cases, supplements can provide the necessary nutrients to bring your body back into balance and prevent potential health problems.

2. Health Conditions and Special Needs

Some health conditions or lifestyle factors can increase the need for specific nutrients. For example:

- **Pregnancy and breastfeeding** : Women who are pregnant or breastfeeding have higher nutrient needs, including folic acid, iron, and calcium.
- **Chronic conditions** : People with chronic conditions such as osteoporosis, diabetes, or digestive disorders may need supplements to help manage their condition and ensure proper nutrient absorption.
- **Age-related needs** : As we age, our bodies absorb nutrients less efficiently. Older adults often need more calcium and vitamin D to support bone health and prevent osteoporosis, as well as B12 to aid cognitive function.

In these cases, a doctor or healthcare professional may recommend specific supplements tailored to the individual's unique needs.

3. Convenience and Time Constraints

In our fast-paced world, preparing a well-balanced meal may not always be practical. For those who don't have time or access to fresh, nutrient-dense foods, supplements can be a quick and easy way to fill gaps. However, supplements should never replace real food, which provides the full spectrum of nutrients and fiber that supplements alone cannot offer.

Sustainable and Natural Supplement Options

As the awareness of health and sustainability grows, many people are turning to natural and sustainable supplement options that align with their values of environmental responsibility. Not all supplements are created equal, and choosing the right ones can make a significant difference in both your health and the planet's well-being.

- **Organic and Whole Food-Based Supplements**

Whole food-based supplements are made from natural, plant-based sources rather than synthetic chemicals. These types of supplements are considered more easily absorbed by the body and are less likely to cause side effects. For example, a whole-food vitamin C supplement made from acerola cherries or rose hips will likely contain a complex of natural bioflavonoids, which work synergistically to enhance absorption and effectiveness.

Organic supplements are also a great option because they're made without the use of synthetic pesticides or fertilizers, which reduces their environmental impact. Choosing organic also ensures that you're supporting farming practices that focus on soil health and biodiversity, which are important for long-term sustainability.

- **Sustainable Sourcing**

Sustainability should also be a top consideration when selecting supplements. Many popular supplements, such as fish oil and certain types of omega-3 fatty acids, come from non-sustainable sources. Overfishing and harmful fishing practices are major threats to marine ecosystems. Therefore, looking for sustainably sourced supplements, such as algae-based omega-3 supplements, is a better alternative for both your health and the planet.

Similarly, look for supplements that are certified by third-party organizations that ensure ethical practices. Certifications such as Fair Trade or Non-GMO Project Verified can help ensure that the supplements you choose are produced responsibly and sustainably.

- **Plant-Based and Vegan Supplements**

For those following a plant-based or vegan diet, finding vegan-friendly supplements is essential. Many vitamins, such as B12 and omega-3, are typically derived from animal products. Fortunately, there are now plant-based alternatives available. For example, B12 supplements can be derived from fermented foods or fortified with synthetic forms of B12 that are suitable for vegans. Plant-based omega-3 supplements, made from algae, provide a sustainable and vegan-friendly alternative to fish-based options.

Additionally, plant-based supplements, such as turmeric, spirulina, or chlorella, offer numerous health benefits while supporting sustainability. These supplements are often cultivated using minimal resources and have a lower environmental impact than conventional supplements.

How to Balance Diet and Supplements for Optimal Health

While supplements can be beneficial in certain circumstances, it's important to remember that they should never replace a balanced, nutrient-dense diet. Ideally, your food should be the primary source of nourishment, as whole foods provide a wide range of nutrients that supplements cannot fully replicate. However, supplements can be useful in certain situations, as long as they are used wisely.

- **Prioritize Whole Foods First**

The first step in maintaining a healthy diet is to prioritize whole, minimally processed foods. Fruits, vegetables, whole grains, legumes, nuts, seeds, and lean proteins are packed with vitamins, minerals, fiber, and antioxidants that promote overall health. A well-rounded diet should provide the majority of the nutrients you need, without the need for supplements.

For example, getting plenty of dark leafy greens, citrus fruits, nuts, and seeds can give you all the vitamin C, calcium, and healthy fats your body needs. Whole grains like quinoa and brown rice provide fiber and essential minerals like magnesium, and legumes can provide high-quality plant protein.

- **Use Supplements as a Support, Not a Substitute**

Supplements should be used as a support to fill in any nutritional gaps that your diet might have. For instance, if you're not getting enough vitamin D due to limited sun exposure, a vitamin D supplement can help fill that gap. Similarly, if your diet lacks adequate omega-3s, adding an algae-based omega-3 supplement can help balance your intake.

Be mindful of dosages and avoid excessive use of any one supplement, as overconsumption of certain vitamins and minerals can cause harmful side effects. It's always best to consult with a healthcare provider or nutritionist before adding new supplements to your routine.

- **Focus on Absorption**

Even if you're eating a healthy diet, nutrient absorption is key. Certain nutrients are better absorbed when taken with specific foods. For instance, fat-soluble vitamins like vitamins A, D, E, and K are better absorbed when consumed with healthy fats, such as olive oil or avocado. Magnesium supplements, on the other hand, are best taken in the evening as they can have a calming effect on the body.

Additionally, some people have impaired digestion or health conditions that reduce nutrient absorption, making supplements necessary to ensure adequate intake of vital nutrients.

Supplements can undoubtedly play a crucial role in supporting health, especially when it comes to addressing specific nutrient deficiencies or enhancing overall well-being. However, they should always be viewed as a complement to—not a substitute for—a well-rounded, nutrient-dense diet. The foundation of good health lies in whole foods—fruits, vegetables, whole grains, legumes, and lean proteins—which provide not only essential vitamins and minerals but also fiber, antioxidants, and other bioactive compounds that supplements alone cannot replicate.

Rather than relying on supplements to "fix" a diet lacking in essential nutrients, it's important to focus on making informed choices that prioritize whole, minimally processed foods first. Supplements should only be considered when they address a specific gap or deficiency that diet alone cannot fulfill. For example, individuals who are unable to get adequate sun exposure may need vitamin D supplementation, or those on plant-based diets may require B12 or omega-3s from algae-based sources.

When choosing supplements, sustainability should be at the forefront of your decision-making process. Opt for products that are responsibly sourced and produced with minimal environmental impact. Many supplements on the market today are derived from plants and animals, so it's essential to choose options that align with your values—whether that's supporting regenerative farming practices, minimizing the depletion of natural resources, or choosing cruelty-free alternatives. Plant-based supplements often provide a cleaner, more sustainable option and can help you align your health journey with your commitment to the planet.

Moreover, choosing supplements that are free from synthetic additives, pesticides, and GMOs can contribute to a more natural, holistic approach to supplementation. By ensuring that what you consume is both beneficial for your body and mindful of the planet's health, you can create a balance between optimal nutrition and environmental stewardship. This approach to supplements ultimately supports not only your personal health but also a more sustainable, harmonious relationship with the world around you.

In the end, a mindful and balanced approach to nutrition is key. By focusing on the nourishing power of whole foods while selectively incorporating natural and sustainable supplements when necessary, you can foster long-term well-being—for yourself and for the environment.

Chapter 21

Eating for Long-Term Wellness

The journey toward long-term wellness is grounded in the food we eat and the habits we form around nutrition. It's easy to think of diet as a short-term goal—such as fitting into a dress for an event or losing weight quickly for the summer—but true wellness is achieved when we shift our focus to a sustainable, long-term approach to eating. Our food choices influence our risk of chronic diseases, shape our energy levels, and even play a role in how we age. In this chapter, we will explore how to build a diet that supports lifelong health, the importance of key lifestyle habits, and how maintaining variety in our diet can lead to lasting well-being.

Building a Diet for Longevity and Disease Prevention

Eating for longevity is about making intentional choices that nourish your body with the right balance of nutrients to not only prevent disease but also promote healthy aging. Research consistently shows that diets abundant in whole, minimally processed foods—such as vibrant fruits, leafy vegetables, whole grains, nutrient-dense nuts and seeds, and heart-healthy legumes—are closely linked to longer lifespans and a significantly reduced risk of chronic conditions like heart disease, type 2 diabetes, and certain cancers.

The foods you choose to fuel your body play a vital role in slowing the aging process and maintaining optimal health over the years. By prioritizing a nutrient-dense, plant-rich diet, you are giving your body the essential vitamins, minerals, antioxidants, and fiber it needs to function at its peak, while simultaneously protecting it from the damaging effects of oxidative stress, inflammation, and cellular damage. The power of whole foods lies in their ability to provide a complex array of nutrients that work synergistically to support every system in the body—from boosting immune function to enhancing brain health and improving digestion.

Incorporating a variety of plant-based foods into your meals not only supports longevity but also fosters a balanced approach to aging, ensuring that you're setting yourself up for a lifetime of health, vitality, and well-being.

To start, it's essential to focus on nutrient-dense foods that provide your body with essential vitamins, minerals, fiber, and antioxidants. These nutrients work together to protect against oxidative stress, inflammation, and cellular damage—key factors in aging and disease development.

1. Fruits and Vegetables: Your Superfoods

Fruits and vegetables are the foundation of a longevity-promoting diet. They are packed with antioxidants, vitamins (such as vitamin C, vitamin A, and folate), minerals (like potassium and magnesium), and fiber. A diverse array of fruits and vegetables not only supports a healthy immune system but also protects against heart disease, stroke, and certain cancers. Aim to eat a rainbow of colors, as each color represents different nutrients that offer unique health benefits. Leafy greens like spinach and kale, for example, are rich in vitamin K and calcium, while bright fruits like berries provide powerful antioxidants that reduce inflammation.

2. Whole Grains and Legumes

Whole grains like oats, quinoa, barley, and brown rice are an excellent source of fiber, B vitamins, and minerals such as iron and magnesium. Unlike refined grains, whole grains retain their bran and germ, which are packed with nutrients that help regulate blood sugar levels, reduce inflammation, and support heart health. Similarly, legumes—such as lentils, beans, and peas—are rich in plant-based protein and fiber. These foods help lower cholesterol, support gut health, and maintain a healthy weight.

3. Healthy Fats

Healthy fats from sources like avocados, nuts, seeds, and olive oil are critical for brain health and the prevention of cardiovascular disease. These fats support healthy cell function, reduce inflammation, and help your body absorb fat-soluble vitamins (like vitamins A, D, E, and K). Omega-3 fatty acids, found in fatty fish like salmon and chia seeds, have also been shown to reduce the risk of heart disease, promote cognitive function, and even protect against depression.

4. Lean Proteins

While plant-based proteins are great, lean animal proteins like fish, chicken, and turkey are also an essential part of a healthy diet when consumed in moderation. These provide your body with the amino acids necessary for muscle repair and tissue growth. However, it's crucial to balance these proteins with plant-based options, as a plant-based diet has been shown to have additional health benefits, including lower blood pressure and reduced risk of heart disease.

Key Lifestyle Habits That Support Lifelong Health

While food is the cornerstone of long-term wellness, it's not the only factor that plays a role. Our lifestyle choices, including physical activity, sleep, stress management, and hydration, all contribute to the way our bodies age and function. Here are a few habits to incorporate into your daily routine to enhance your diet and support a healthy life.

1. Regular Physical Activity

Exercise is a key factor in preventing disease and supporting longevity. It promotes cardiovascular health, strengthens bones and muscles, improves mental health, and even helps regulate metabolism and insulin sensitivity. Studies show that people who are physically active have a lower risk of chronic diseases like diabetes, heart disease, and certain cancers. Aim for a mix of aerobic exercise (like walking, running, or cycling) and strength training (like weightlifting or yoga) to support a balanced, well-rounded fitness routine.

2. Quality Sleep

Getting enough sleep is vital for maintaining good health throughout your life. Sleep helps your body repair cells, regulate hormones, and process information. Chronic sleep deprivation has been linked to an increased risk of obesity, diabetes, heart disease, and even early mortality. Aim for 7-9 hours of sleep per night, and establish a regular sleep routine that allows your body to rest and recover fully. Sleep is essential for both physical and mental well-being.

3. Stress Management

Chronic stress can have a significant impact on your health. It can increase inflammation, raise blood pressure, and negatively affect your immune system. Managing stress is critical for long-term wellness. Techniques like meditation, mindfulness, yoga, deep breathing, and even regular hobbies can help lower stress levels and promote emotional health. Make time for self-care and relaxation to balance the pressures of daily life.

4. Staying Hydrated

Water is essential for nearly every function in the body, from regulating temperature to aiding digestion and supporting joint health. Staying hydrated also helps maintain healthy skin and promotes optimal brain function. Aim to drink at least 8 cups of water a day, and more if you are physically active or in hot climates. Herbal teas and water-rich foods like cucumbers and watermelon can also help you stay hydrated.

The Importance of Variety in Your Diet

While it's tempting to stick to a few favorite meals, variety is key to ensuring that you're getting a wide range of nutrients to support long-term health. Different foods provide different vitamins, minerals, and other nutrients, so rotating foods and introducing new ingredients into your meals can fill any potential gaps in your nutrition.

1. Preventing Nutrient Deficiencies

No single food can meet all of your body's nutritional needs, which is why diversity in your diet is essential for long-term wellness. Our bodies thrive on a variety of vitamins, minerals, proteins, and other nutrients, each contributing to different physiological processes. For instance, while fruits and vegetables like leafy greens are packed with antioxidants, fiber, and vitamin K, they might lack sufficient protein or certain essential fats. Including a wide range of food sources in your diet, both plant-based and animal-based, ensures that you're covering all the necessary bases for optimal health.

Take vitamin B12, for example. This vital nutrient, crucial for brain health and the production of red blood cells, is primarily found in animal products such as eggs, meat, and dairy. While leafy greens are rich in vitamin K, they won't provide enough vitamin B12 on their own. By complementing plant-based foods with nutrient-dense animal products or fortified plant foods, you can ensure you're getting a balance of vitamins and minerals. Whole grains and legumes are also powerful allies in providing protein and other essential nutrients like iron and magnesium, which are important for muscle function, energy, and bone health.

Furthermore, variety allows you to experience the health benefits of different food groups and prevents nutrient gaps. By including a mix of different fruits, vegetables, grains, legumes, nuts, seeds, and lean proteins, you're providing your body with everything it needs to function efficiently and prevent nutritional deficiencies. This diverse intake helps manage inflammation, supports heart health, stabilizes blood sugar, and strengthens the immune system, all of which play critical roles in disease prevention and longevity.

It's important to view food as a tool for long-term health, rather than focusing on short-term or restrictive trends. Making conscious, balanced choices, whether plant-based or animal-based, is an investment in your wellness. By aiming for variety and nutrient-rich, whole foods, you set the stage for a healthier, longer life. This approach fosters not only a well-balanced diet but also a sustainable lifestyle that can support your health for years to come.

2. Supporting Gut Health

Your gut health depends on the diversity of foods you eat. A diverse diet introduces a variety of fibers, prebiotics, and probiotics to the gut, which support the healthy bacteria living there. These bacteria are essential for digestion, nutrient absorption, and immune function. Incorporating a mix of fiber-rich foods, fermented foods, and plant-based options can help nourish your gut microbiome and promote overall well-being.

3. Keeping Meals Exciting

Eating the same foods repeatedly can make meals feel dull and uninspiring. By experimenting with new ingredients and flavors, you keep mealtime interesting while benefiting from the wide range of nutrients they offer. A colorful, varied plate not only supports your health but also enhances your relationship with food by making eating an enjoyable experience.

Conclusion

Eating for long-term wellness is about cultivating a lifestyle that promotes health, vitality, and sustainability over time. It's not about chasing the next trendy diet or making drastic changes that are unsustainable; it's about adopting habits that nourish your body, mind, and the planet for the long haul. By prioritizing whole, nutrient-dense foods, staying active, managing stress effectively, and ensuring that your diet includes a variety of foods, you can not only improve your quality of life but also boost your chances of living a longer, more vibrant existence.

One of the key principles of long-term wellness is variety. Our bodies thrive on diversity, and no single food can meet all our nutritional needs. By eating a wide range of plant-based and animal-based foods, we provide our bodies with the essential vitamins, minerals, protein, and fats required for optimal health. A varied diet supports everything from a strong immune system and healthy digestion to heart health and mental clarity. The more diverse your meals, the more you ensure you're getting the full spectrum of nutrients your body needs to function at its best.

But wellness isn't just about what you eat; it's also about how you live. Maintaining an active lifestyle, managing stress, and ensuring quality sleep all play crucial roles in how we feel on a day-to-day basis and in our long-term health. Regular exercise boosts mood, supports metabolism, reduces the risk of chronic diseases, and improves overall longevity. Mindful stress management techniques like meditation or yoga can lower cortisol levels, prevent burnout, and improve mental clarity, allowing you to be present in your daily life. And don't forget about sleep! It's when our bodies repair and rejuvenate, making it just as important as what we eat or how much we move.

Eating for long-term wellness is about seeing the big picture—it's about understanding that every meal and every habit you choose has the power to either support or undermine your health. The decisions you make today not only impact your personal well-being, but they also contribute to the broader health of the environment. By choosing more plant-based foods, reducing food waste, and being mindful of where and how your food is sourced, you're playing a role in promoting a more sustainable food system for generations to come.

As we embrace these intentional choices, we help create a ripple effect that touches every aspect of our lives—from the food systems that sustain us to the communities we build and the planet we inhabit. The changes we make today will lay the groundwork for a future that is healthier, happier, and more harmonious. Through mindful eating, conscious living, and collective action, we can set the stage for a future where personal wellness and planetary health are inextricably linked.

Ultimately, the journey toward long-term wellness is a process of ongoing self-care and mindful choices. It's about making small, intentional decisions each day that add up to significant, lasting change. As we embrace these practices, we align our daily actions with our values, ensuring that we're not only nurturing ourselves but also caring for the world around us. The foundation we build today will lead to a more resilient and thriving future, both for our bodies and the planet. Through the Food Revolution, we can transform the way we eat, the way we live, and the way we contribute to the world, creating a legacy of health, sustainability, and well-being for future generations.

Chapter 22

Creating a Sustainable Eating Lifestyle for Your Family

Sustainable eating isn't just a lifestyle choice—it's a collective commitment that can transform the way your entire family nourishes itself and interacts with the world. When you make sustainable eating a family practice, you're not only promoting better health for everyone but also helping reduce your environmental impact, create lasting habits, and instill important values in your children. This is an opportunity to teach your kids about the profound connection between the food they eat and the planet they live on.

The beauty of sustainable eating lies in its ability to adapt to different stages of life. Whether you're planning meals for toddlers, teenagers, or adults, creating a balanced approach that aligns with everyone's nutritional needs and tastes is not only achievable but rewarding. By integrating sustainable practices into your family's routine—such as making informed food choices, prioritizing plant-based meals, and reducing waste—you'll cultivate a healthier household while positively impacting the environment.

In this chapter, we'll explore how to craft a sustainable eating lifestyle that works for everyone in your family, regardless of age or preference. We'll share practical strategies for encouraging kids to embrace healthy, sustainable foods, introduce fun and creative meal planning ideas that engage the whole family, and offer family-friendly recipes that are both nourishing and planet-friendly. By working together in the kitchen, involving children in meal prep, and making food choices as a family, you'll not only create stronger bonds but also lay the foundation for long-term healthy habits.

Sustainable eating can be easy, enjoyable, and deeply fulfilling. The goal is to make it a seamless part of your family's everyday life, so that your children grow up with a solid understanding of how their food choices affect their health and the world around them. Through small changes, thoughtful planning, and a shared commitment to doing better, you can make a big difference—one meal at a time.

How to Make Sustainable Eating Work for All Ages

One of the most important aspects of creating a sustainable eating lifestyle for your family is making sure it works for everyone, regardless of age or dietary needs. Sustainability doesn't have to be difficult, and it's important to make small, gradual changes that the whole family can embrace. Here are some key ways to make sustainable eating work for all ages:

- **Start With Small, Manageable Changes:** The idea of switching to a fully sustainable lifestyle might seem overwhelming at first, especially for families with young children or picky eaters. It's important to take gradual steps to make the transition easier. Begin by making small, manageable changes like reducing the consumption of single-use plastic packaging, choosing more plant-based meals, and buying seasonal, local produce. Slowly build these habits into your family's daily routine so it feels natural rather than forced.

- **Involve the Entire Family in Meal Planning:** When transitioning to a more sustainable diet, it's essential to involve everyone in the family. Talk to your kids about the importance of sustainability, and get their input on what meals they would enjoy. This can help them feel more invested in the process and encourage them to make healthier choices. Depending on their age, allow your children to help pick out groceries, prepare meals, and try new ingredients. Giving them ownership over what they eat can make them more likely to embrace sustainable eating habits.

- **Focus on Flexibility, Not Perfection:** It's important to remember that adopting a sustainable lifestyle doesn't have to be all-or-nothing. Sustainability is about making conscious, intentional choices that add up over time. If your family occasionally eats out, or if there's a special event that involves less sustainable options, don't stress. The goal is to make consistent efforts toward sustainability, not to achieve perfection.

- **Plan for Special Dietary Needs:** For families with specific dietary restrictions or preferences (such as gluten-free, dairy-free, or vegetarian), it's crucial to create a meal plan that works for everyone. Sustainable eating can be adapted to meet all types of dietary needs. For example, choosing plant-based options can benefit those who follow vegetarian or vegan diets, and gluten-free families can still prioritize local, organic foods. Adapt sustainable principles to your family's unique needs while still focusing on reducing environmental impact.

Tips for Encouraging Kids to Eat Healthy, Sustainable Foods

Getting kids to eat healthy, sustainable foods can be challenging, especially if they're used to processed snacks or fast food. However, with a little creativity and patience, it's entirely possible to get your kids excited about eating sustainably. Here are some tips to encourage your children to eat healthier, more sustainable foods:

- **Lead by Example:** Children are more likely to adopt healthy habits when they see their parents practicing them. Make sure that you are setting a good example by choosing sustainable foods for yourself. Show your kids how eating plant-based meals, locally sourced foods, and whole ingredients can be delicious and fun. When they see you enjoying healthy, sustainable food, they're more likely to follow suit.

- **Make Healthy Foods Fun:** Presentation is key when it comes to getting kids excited about food. Try making healthy meals colorful, fun, and interactive. Create a "build-your-own" meal bar with toppings for tacos, wraps, or bowls that allow kids to customize their meals with fresh vegetables, proteins, and whole grains. Use cookie cutters to make fruits and vegetables fun shapes, or involve them in preparing meals so they feel like they have some control over what they eat.

- **Educate Them About Sustainability:** It's never too early to teach children about sustainability and why it matters. Explain to them how choosing sustainable foods helps protect the environment and improves health. You could read books or watch videos about the importance of food systems, agriculture, and the impact of food waste. By making sustainability part of the conversation, you empower kids to make thoughtful choices and become more mindful of their food consumption.

- **Get Them Involved in the Kitchen:** Kids love to help in the kitchen, and involving them in meal prep is a great way to get them more interested in eating healthy foods. Let your children help chop vegetables, mix ingredients, or assemble dishes. The more involved they are in preparing their meals, the more likely they are to appreciate the food and be excited to eat it. This also teaches them valuable cooking skills and helps them feel more in control of their eating habits.

- **Make Healthy Snacks Easily Accessible:** Kids often snack throughout the day, so make it easy for them to choose healthy options. Stock up on fresh fruits, veggies, nuts, seeds, and whole grain snacks. Pre-cut fruits and vegetables and place them in easy-to-reach containers for quick access. The easier it is for your kids to grab healthy snacks, the more likely they will choose them over less nutritious options.

Meal Planning and Family-Friendly Sustainable Recipes

Meal planning is a key component of sustainable eating. By planning your meals ahead of time, you can ensure that you're making the most of your ingredients, minimizing food waste, and creating balanced meals that work for your entire family. Below are some strategies for meal planning and some family-friendly, sustainable recipes that can help make this process easier:

- **Plan Your Meals Around Seasonal, Local Ingredients:** When creating your meal plan, choose recipes that highlight seasonal fruits, vegetables, and other locally sourced ingredients. Local produce is often fresher, more nutritious, and has a lower environmental impact due to reduced transportation. Take a trip to your local farmers' market or join a community-supported agriculture (CSA) program to discover what's in season and plan your meals accordingly.

- **Batch Cooking and Leftovers:** Batch cooking is an excellent way to reduce food waste while saving time and energy. Prepare larger portions of meals that can be enjoyed throughout the week, like soups, stews, casseroles, or grain bowls. Leftovers can be repurposed into new meals, reducing food waste and maximizing your ingredients.
- **Make Simple, Nutritious Meals:** Family-friendly meals don't have to be complicated. Focus on simple, nutritious meals that are easy to prepare and use a variety of plant-based and sustainable ingredients. Here are a few sustainable recipes your family can enjoy together:

1. **Vegetable Stir-Fry:** A quick and easy dish that's loaded with colorful, seasonal vegetables. Serve it over brown rice or quinoa for a hearty, nutritious meal. Add tofu or tempeh for protein, and top with a simple homemade stir-fry sauce made with soy sauce, garlic, ginger, and sesame oil.
2. **Lentil Tacos:** A delicious and plant-based alternative to traditional meat tacos. Cook lentils with onions, garlic, and spices (such as cumin, paprika, and chili powder) and serve in soft corn tortillas with fresh toppings like avocado, salsa, and shredded lettuce.
3. **Roasted Root Vegetables and Quinoa Bowl:** A hearty, satisfying dish perfect for fall and winter. Roast root vegetables like sweet potatoes, carrots, and beets, and serve them with cooked quinoa. Top with a lemon-tahini dressing and some toasted nuts or seeds for crunch.

4. **Chickpea Salad:** A refreshing, protein-packed salad that's perfect for a light lunch or dinner. Toss together chickpeas, cucumber, cherry tomatoes, red onion, and leafy greens, and dress with olive oil, lemon juice, and herbs like parsley and dill.
5. **Veggie-Packed Pasta:** A simple pasta dish that incorporates lots of fresh veggies like zucchini, bell peppers, and spinach. Toss with a marinara sauce made from canned tomatoes, garlic, and olive oil. Add some plant-based protein like lentils or beans, and sprinkle with nutritional yeast for a cheesy flavor.

Creating a sustainable eating lifestyle for your family is not just about making one-time decisions—it's about cultivating a mindset and setting a foundation that will benefit both your health and the environment for years to come. Achieving this involves thoughtful planning, creativity, and a commitment to long-term, healthy choices. When you actively involve your children in the process, you not only empower them to make better food decisions but also teach them valuable life lessons about sustainability, responsibility, and the importance of mindful consumption.

Leading by example is one of the most powerful tools in shaping your family's eating habits. When your children see you making thoughtful food choices, prioritizing fresh, whole foods, and showing care for the planet, they are more likely to adopt similar habits themselves. By making small, manageable changes in your grocery shopping, meal preparation, and waste reduction practices, you can gradually shift toward a more sustainable way of eating without overwhelming your family.

Meal planning plays a significant role in creating a sustainable eating lifestyle. It allows you to shop with intention, reduce food waste, and ensure that each meal contributes to your family's well-being. Cooking together as a family further strengthens the bond, while also providing an opportunity to teach kids about where their food comes from, how to make nutritious meals, and the joy of preparing food from scratch. From planting a small vegetable garden to preparing simple, plant-based meals, there are countless ways to make sustainable eating fun, practical, and rewarding for every family member.

Sustainable eating is not a one-size-fits-all approach, and it doesn't require perfection. Small steps can lead to big changes, and over time, those changes can have a lasting impact on your family's health and the planet. By embracing sustainable food choices, your family can build a healthier, happier future while also contributing to the preservation of our environment for generations to come.

Chapter 23

The Future of Food: Embracing a New Way to Eat

As global challenges such as climate change, over consumption of resources, and an ever-expanding population become more pressing, the future of food is being reshaped to address these critical issues. How we produce food, the types of foods we consume, and the way we manage food waste are now central to creating a more sustainable and healthier food system. In the past, food choices were primarily motivated by taste, tradition, or convenience, but today, we must also make decisions that take into account the broader environmental and health implications. What we eat today will have a lasting impact on our planet tomorrow.

This chapter will delve into the emerging trends in sustainable food systems that are leading the way toward a more resilient and responsible food future. These trends are not simply theoretical but are becoming integral parts of our food systems—whether it's the rise of plant-based diets, the shift toward regenerative agriculture, or the growing focus on food sovereignty. We'll also explore how technological innovations are accelerating these changes. Technologies such as vertical farming, precision agriculture, lab-grown meat, and sustainable packaging solutions are revolutionizing how we grow, distribute, and consume food. These innovations present promising solutions that aim to minimize environmental impact, improve food accessibility, and support local economies.

However, while technological advances are crucial, we cannot overlook the power of individual actions. The choices we make as consumers—what we eat, how we shop, and how we dispose of food—play a critical role in driving the transformation of the food system. In this chapter, we'll offer practical advice for continuing your journey toward a healthier, more sustainable diet. Simple actions like reducing food waste, supporting sustainable brands, buying locally, and adopting mindful eating habits can help create a ripple effect that extends far beyond your own kitchen.

The future of food is a collective effort, one that requires collaboration between individuals, communities, industries, and governments. But together, we can forge a future where food nourishes not only our bodies but also the planet. Embracing a more sustainable food system is essential for the well-being of both people and the environment. By understanding and acting on these emerging trends and innovations, we can all play a part in shaping a food system that is equitable, sustainable, and capable of meeting the needs of generations to come.

Emerging Trends in Sustainable Food Systems

The concept of sustainable food systems is gaining traction as individuals, communities, and organizations around the globe recognize the importance of aligning food production with ecological, economic, and social sustainability. This new way of thinking about food transcends traditional agricultural models and focuses on the long-term health of the planet as well as the people who depend on it for nourishment.

One of the most significant trends in sustainable food systems is the move toward plant-based diets. As concerns about the environmental impact of animal agriculture grow, plant-based eating is emerging as a key solution for reducing our ecological footprint. The livestock industry is a major contributor to greenhouse gas emissions, land degradation, deforestation, and water pollution. By shifting to plant-based foods, such as fruits, vegetables, grains, legumes, and nuts, individuals can help mitigate climate change and reduce strain on the planet's natural resources.

In addition to plant-based eating, the concept of regenerative agriculture is gaining momentum. Regenerative agriculture focuses on improving soil health, increasing biodiversity, and capturing carbon in the soil through practices like crop rotation, agroforestry, and no-till farming. This method of farming aims to restore the health of the land rather than depleting it, creating a more sustainable and resilient food system for future generations.

Another emerging trend is the rise of vertical farming and urban agriculture. These methods of food production involve growing crops in controlled, indoor environments or urban spaces, which helps to reduce the environmental impact of traditional farming methods. Vertical farms use less land, water, and energy compared to conventional agriculture, and they often grow crops closer to urban centers, reducing food miles and the carbon footprint associated with transportation.

Finally, there is a growing focus on local and seasonal food sourcing. With an increasing awareness of the environmental costs associated with food production and transportation, many consumers are turning to local farmers and markets to source fresh, seasonal produce. Buying locally not only supports the local economy but also reduces the carbon footprint of food by minimizing the distance it must travel to reach consumers.

The Role of Technology and Innovation in Sustainable Eating

As we move toward a more sustainable food system, technology and innovation are playing a crucial role in reshaping the way we produce, distribute, and consume food. Advances in agricultural technology, food production, and sustainable packaging are helping create more efficient, eco-friendly systems.

One of the most exciting innovations in sustainable food production is lab-grown or cultured meat. Lab-grown meat is produced by cultivating animal cells in a lab setting, offering the potential for meat production without the environmental costs associated with traditional livestock farming. Cultured meat could significantly reduce the land, water, and energy used in meat production, as well as eliminate the greenhouse gas emissions that result from raising and slaughtering animals.

Another groundbreaking development in sustainable food technology is the rise of plant-based meat alternatives. Companies like Beyond Meat and Impossible Foods have pioneered plant-based burgers, sausages, and other meat substitutes that closely mimic the taste, texture, and appearance of real meat. These products offer a more sustainable alternative to traditional meat by using plant ingredients to replicate the nutritional profile and sensory experience of animal-based foods. By replacing animal products with plant-based alternatives, consumers can reduce their environmental impact while still enjoying the flavors and experiences associated with meat.

Precision agriculture is also making waves in sustainable food production. This technology uses data and analytics to optimize farming practices, reduce waste, and minimize the environmental footprint of agriculture. For example, sensors and drones can monitor soil health, water usage, and crop conditions, helping farmers make more informed decisions and reduce their reliance on pesticides, fertilizers, and water. By increasing efficiency and reducing resource use, precision agriculture has the potential to make food production more sustainable and resilient in the face of climate change.

Sustainable packaging is another area where innovation is having a significant impact. With the growing problem of plastic waste, companies are developing new, eco-friendly packaging solutions to reduce the environmental burden of packaging materials. Biodegradable packaging, edible packaging, and reusable containers are all part of the move toward reducing single-use plastics in the food industry. In addition, food waste is being repurposed into packaging materials, with innovations like fungi-based packaging and algae-based plastics helping to reduce reliance on fossil fuels and synthetic materials.

In the digital realm, the rise of food apps and platforms that promote sustainable eating is helping consumers make informed decisions about what they buy and eat. Apps that provide information on food sourcing, carbon footprints, and food waste are helping people better understand the environmental impact of their food choices and encouraging them to make more sustainable decisions. Additionally, apps that help individuals track their food waste and provide tips on reducing it can help households minimize food waste and save money in the process.

Continuing Your Journey Toward a Healthier, More Sustainable Future

As we move into the future of food, each of us has an important role to play in shaping a more sustainable and healthy food system. While larger systemic changes are necessary to address global challenges, individual actions can collectively make a significant impact.

One of the best ways to continue your journey toward a healthier, more sustainable future is by educating yourself and others about the environmental and health benefits of sustainable eating. By staying informed about the latest trends in food systems, sustainability practices, and emerging technologies, you can make better decisions about the food you buy and eat.

Another important step is to make small, sustainable changes to your diet. Start by reducing your meat and dairy consumption, experimenting with plant-based alternatives, and incorporating more locally grown, seasonal produce into your meals. Reducing food waste is also a key aspect of sustainable eating—plan your meals, store food properly, and get creative with leftovers to minimize waste.

Support local farmers and sustainable food businesses by buying directly from them or through community-supported agriculture (CSA) programs. These initiatives promote sustainable farming practices and help create stronger, more resilient local food systems. By supporting sustainable food sources, you contribute to the overall health and longevity of the food system and the environment.

Incorporate sustainable food choices into your daily routine by making eco-friendly packaging choices, reducing single-use plastics, and composting food scraps. Composting not only reduces waste but also helps return valuable nutrients to the soil, supporting healthy ecosystems and improving soil quality.

Lastly, engage in conversations about food sustainability within your community. Advocate for policies that support sustainable farming, food access, and waste reduction. By raising awareness and encouraging others to make sustainable food choices, we can collectively create a more sustainable future.

The future of food is not just about what we eat, but how we produce and consume it. With a growing awareness of the environmental and health challenges tied to our current food system, there is a collective push toward more sustainable, equitable, and healthier alternatives. From plant-based diets to regenerative agriculture, emerging trends are reshaping the way we think about food. These changes are not just a passing trend; they represent a fundamental shift in how we feed the world in a way that is better for the planet, better for our communities, and better for our health.

As we look to the future, technology and innovation are playing a key role in driving this transformation. Advances in food science, sustainable farming practices, and new food production methods like vertical farming and lab-grown meat are all making it possible to meet the growing demand for food while minimizing our environmental footprint. These innovations offer exciting opportunities to not only make our food system more sustainable but also to improve the quality and accessibility of food for all.

The future of food is also about rethinking the way we interact with the food we consume. By embracing mindful eating practices, being more conscious of food waste, and supporting local, sustainable food systems, we can all contribute to a more resilient food culture. This shift is not just about personal choices but about coming together as a global community to address the challenges of climate change, food security, and public health.

We have the power to shape a future where food nourishes not just our bodies, but the world around us. The decisions we make today will impact generations to come, and the future of food is in our hands. By adopting a more sustainable, healthy, and conscious approach to eating, we can build a food system that benefits everyone —from the farmers and workers who grow our food to the communities who enjoy it, and ultimately, to the planet itself. Together, we can embrace a new way of eating—one that is not only good for us but also good for the Earth, ensuring that the future of food is one of balance, health, and sustainability.

Chapter 24

Conclusion

Your Food Revolution Starts Today

The journey toward a healthier and more sustainable way of eating begins with a single step. It starts with the food choices we make every day—choices that have the potential to improve our personal health and contribute to the well-being of the planet. If there is one thing to take away from this book, it's that food matters—not just for our bodies, but for the environment, too.

In the chapters that followed, we've explored various aspects of healthy, sustainable eating. From understanding the importance of nutrition to learning how to reduce food waste, we've covered the essential components of making informed food choices. Along the way, we've discovered that even small changes can have a lasting impact when it comes to both personal health and environmental sustainability.

Now, it's time for you to take the next step. The Food Revolution doesn't require radical changes overnight, but rather a commitment to being more mindful, intentional, and conscious about what we put on our plates. Whether it's reducing your carbon footprint by incorporating more plant-based meals into your diet, cutting down on food waste, or simply becoming more aware of where your food comes from, each action counts.

Remember, the goal isn't to achieve perfection. You don't have to make every meal 100% sustainable or healthy right away. Instead, think of your journey as an evolving process. Each meal is an opportunity to make better choices. Some days you'll succeed, and other days you'll slip up—but that's okay. What matters most is that you're taking steps in the right direction.

Be proud of every small change you make. Whether it's swapping out a processed snack for a piece of fresh fruit, supporting local farmers, or committing to composting your food scraps, each of these actions plays a role in the bigger picture. The choices you make today have the power to shape a better tomorrow—for you, for your community, and for the planet.

Resources for Continued Learning

While this book provides you with the foundational knowledge and tools to get started on your food revolution, the journey doesn't end here. There are countless resources available that can help you deepen your understanding of healthy, sustainable eating and continue your growth along the way.

Here are some recommended resources for continued learning:

1. **Books:**
    - *The Omnivore's Dilemma* by Michael Pollan: This book takes a deep dive into the food system, exploring the origins of the food we eat and its impact on our health and the environment.
    - *How to Be a Conscious Eater* by Sophie Egan: A practical guide for navigating modern food choices with an emphasis on health and sustainability.

- *Eating on the Wild Side* by Jo Robinson: Learn about the nutritional benefits of consuming whole, natural foods and how to make the best choices for both health and the environment.

3. **Websites:**
    - **The Environmental Working Group (EWG):** Offers tips on reducing pesticide use and making more sustainable food choices. (www.ewg.org)
    - **The Food and Agriculture Organization (FAO):** Provides reports and resources on sustainable agriculture and global food systems. (www.fao.org)
    - **The Plant-Based Dietitian:** Offers advice, recipes, and information on transitioning to a plant-based diet while meeting nutritional needs. (www.plantbaseddietitian.com)

5. **Documentaries and Films:**
    - *Forks Over Knives* : A compelling documentary on the benefits of a whole-food, plant-based diet for both personal health and the environment.
    - *The Game Changers* : This film examines the benefits of plant-based eating for athletic performance and overall health.
    - *The True Cost* : A documentary that explores the environmental and social costs of the global fashion industry, offering valuable insights into sustainable consumer choices.

7. **Podcasts:**
    - **The Minimalist Vegan Podcast:** Discussions on how to live a simpler, more sustainable life, with a focus on plant-based eating.

- **The Sustainable Dish Podcast:** A podcast that covers topics related to nutrition, farming, sustainability, and animal welfare.
- **The Food Revolution Network Podcast:** Offers expert interviews and insights into healthy eating, food systems, and sustainability.

9. **Online Courses:**
    - **Coursera – Sustainable Food Systems:** An online course exploring food systems and their environmental impact, taught by experts in the field.
    - **Plant-Based Nutrition Course (eCornell):** A deep dive into plant-based nutrition, offering evidence-based information on the health benefits of a plant-based diet.
    - **FutureLearn – Eating for the Environment:** An online course that explores how our food choices can help build a more sustainable future.

11. **Local Community Resources:**
    - Many local farmers' markets, co-ops, and food banks offer educational programs on sustainable eating, composting, and reducing food waste. Check out these resources in your community for hands-on learning and direct engagement with local producers.
    - **Sustainable Agriculture Networks:** Joining local groups focused on sustainable farming and eating practices can be a great way to get involved and learn from others.

Building a Supportive Community for Healthy, Sustainable Eating

One of the most powerful ways to maintain motivation and stay committed to a healthier, more sustainable food lifestyle is by surrounding yourself with like-minded individuals. Building a supportive community can provide the encouragement and inspiration needed to stay on track and take action.

Here are some ways to find or create a community of individuals who share your passion for healthy, sustainable eating:

1. **Join Online Communities:**
   - Many online groups and forums are dedicated to topics like plant-based eating, sustainability, and food waste reduction. Platforms like Facebook, Reddit, and Instagram offer plenty of places to connect with others, share tips, recipes, and experiences, and ask questions when you're stuck.

3. **Attend Local Events and Workshops:**
   - Look for events in your community, such as cooking classes, nutrition workshops, or sustainability conferences. These are great opportunities to learn from experts, meet new people, and deepen your knowledge.

5. **Start a Meal Planning Group:**
   - Organize a group of friends or family to join you in planning and prepping meals together. This can be a fun and supportive way to share recipes, reduce waste, and stay motivated.

7. **Volunteer with Local Organizations:**
   - Many non-profits and local organizations focus on food insecurity, sustainable agriculture, and

environmental protection. Volunteering can help you connect with others who share your commitment to making a positive impact.

9. **Support Local Food Initiatives:**
    ◦ Whether it's supporting local farmers or engaging in community gardening, becoming active in your local food system can help foster connections with those who are also interested in creating a healthier, more sustainable food culture.

Your Food Revolution Starts Today

The journey toward a healthier and more sustainable way of eating starts now. The choices you make today, whether it's opting for plant-based meals, reducing food waste, or supporting sustainable farming practices, have the power to create lasting change. While it may seem overwhelming at times, remember that every small action counts.

By taking the first step today, you're not just changing your own habits—you're becoming part of a movement that has the potential to transform the future of food. So, as you begin this journey, take a moment to appreciate the impact of your choices and commit to making those changes with intention and confidence.

The Food Revolution is waiting for you. Are you ready to join?

Chapter 25

References

Chapter 3 - 4:

1. National Institutes of Health (NIH). "Protein and Health Professional." U.S. Department of Health and Human Services, 2021.
2. Harvard T.H. Chan School of Public Health. "Fats and Health." 2022.
3. American Heart Association. "Carbohydrates." 2020.
4. National Institutes of Health (NIH). "Vitamins and Minerals." U.S. Department of Health and Human Services, 2020.
5. Mayo Clinic. "Fiber: How Much Do You Need Every Day?" Mayo Foundation for Medical Education and Research, 2021.
6. National Institutes of Health (NIH). "Whole Grains and Health." U.S. Department of Health and Human Services, 2020.
7. Harvard T.H. Chan School of Public Health. "The Nutrition Source: Vegetables and Fruits." 2021.
8. American Heart Association. "The Benefits of Eating Whole Grains." 2021.

Chapter 5:

- National Institutes of Health (NIH). "Climate Change and Agriculture: Impacts and Opportunities."
- Harvard T.H. Chan School of Public Health. "Plant-Based Diets and Sustainability."

- American Heart Association. "The Environmental Impact of Food Choices."
- Food and Agriculture Organization (FAO). "Global Food Waste Statistics and Mitigation Strategies."
- United Nations Environment Programme (UNEP). "Sustainable Consumption and Production Patterns."

Chapter 6 :

- National Institutes of Health (NIH). "Environmental Impact of Food Production."
- Harvard T.H. Chan School of Public Health. "Plant-Based Diets and Sustainability."
- Food and Agriculture Organization (FAO). "Livestock's Long Shadow."
- United Nations Environment Programme (UNEP). "Sustainable Food Systems and Biodiversity."
- American Heart Association. "Water Use and Agriculture."

Chapter 7 :

- U.S. Food and Drug Administration (FDA), "A Guide to Nutrition Labeling."
- Food and Agriculture Organization (FAO), "Sustainable Food Systems and Certification."
- USDA National Organic Program, "Organic Certification Standards."
- The Non-GMO Project, "Understanding Non-GMO Certification."
- Fairtrade International, "The Benefits of Fair Trade Certification."

Chapter 8 :

- Food and Agriculture Organization (FAO). "Sustainable Food Systems and Agriculture."
- Environmental Working Group (EWG). "Clean Fifteen & Dirty Dozen: A Guide to Pesticides in Produce."
- The Organic Center. "Benefits of Organic Agriculture."
- USDA. "Food Waste Reduction and Sustainability."
- Harvard T.H. Chan School of Public Health. "Sustainable Eating and Food Choices."

Chapter 9 :

- National Institutes of Health (NIH). "Healthy Eating."
- Harvard T.H. Chan School of Public Health. "The Nutrition Source."
- U.S. Environmental Protection Agency (EPA). "Reducing Wasted Food."
- USDA. "MyPlate: A Guide to Healthy Eating."
- Food and Agriculture Organization (FAO). "Food Loss and Waste."

Chapter 10 :

- "The China Study" by T. Colin Campbell and Thomas M. Campbell
- "How Not to Die" by Michael Greger
- American Heart Association - "Plant-Based Diets"
- "The Forks Over Knives Plan" by Alona Pulde and Matthew Lederman

- Physicians Committee for Responsible Medicine
- Food and Agriculture Organization (FAO) - "The Role of Animal Products in the Global Food System"
- National Institutes of Health (NIH) - Office of Dietary Supplements

Chapter 11 :

- "Nutritional Guidelines for a Healthy Diet," Harvard T.H. Chan School of Public Health.
- "Protein and Amino Acids," National Institutes of Health.
- "The Role of Red Meat in a Healthy Diet," American Heart Association.
- "Zinc and Health," National Institutes of Health.
- "Iron: Fact Sheet for Health Professionals," National Institutes of Health.
- "B12 and Veganism," The Vegetarian Resource Group.
- "Saturated Fat and Cardiovascular Disease," American Heart Association.

Chapter 12 :

- "The Energy Efficiency of Cooking Appliances." Energy.gov.
- "The Benefits of Plant-Based Eating for Health and the Environment." World Health Organization.
- "Sustainable Cooking Practices." Environmental Protection Agency (EPA).
- "Roasting Vegetables: Benefits and Tips." Harvard T.H. Chan School of Public Health.

- "Cooking Methods and Nutrient Retention." National Institutes of Health.
- "Reducing Food Waste at Home." United Nations Environment Programme.

Chapter 13 :
- "The Plant-Based Dietitian" by Julieanna Hever
- Environmental Working Group (EWG) – "Dirty Dozen and Clean Fifteen"
- "How to Cook Everything" by Mark Bittman
- USDA – "Budget-Friendly Meal Planning"
- "The Sustainable Food Handbook" by Anastasia L. L.

Chapter 14 :
- "The Omnivore's Dilemma" by Michael Pollan
- Food and Agriculture Organization (FAO) - "The State of Food and Agriculture"
- Environmental Working Group (EWG) - "Meat Eater's Guide to Climate Change + Health"
- "Eating on the Wild Side" by Jo Robinson
- United Nations Environment Programme (UNEP) - "Sustainable Diets"

Chapter 15 :
- Food and Agriculture Organization of the United Nations (FAO) – Reports on global food waste and its impact.
- Environmental Protection Agency (EPA) – Guidelines for composting and reducing waste.
- National Resources Defense Council (NRDC) – Studies and strategies on food waste reduction.

- Zero Waste International Alliance – Tips for achieving a zero-waste lifestyle.
- Books: *Waste-Free Kitchen Handbook* by Dana Gunders and *Composting for a New Generation* by Michelle Balz.

Chapter 16 :

- "Mindful Eating: A Guide to Rediscovering a Healthy and Joyful Relationship with Food" by Jan Chozen Bays
- "The Power of Habit: Why We Do What We Do in Life and Business" by Charles Duhigg
- "Emotional Eating: A Practical Guide to Break Free from Unhealthy Eating Habits" by Eva Ritvo
- "The Plant-Based Diet for Beginners: 75 Delicious, Healthy Whole-Food Recipes" by Gabriel Miller

Chapter 17 :

- Kabat-Zinn, J. (1990). *Full Catastrophe Living: Using the Wisdom of Your Body and Mind to Face Stress, Pain, and Illness* . Delta.
- Kristeller, J. L., & Wolever, R. Q. (2011). Mindfulness-based eating awareness training for treating binge eating disorder: The conceptual foundation. *Eating Disorders* , 19(1), 49-61.
- Tapper, K., & Murphy, S. (2019). Mindful eating: An intervention for the prevention of overeating and obesity. *International Journal of Behavioral Nutrition and Physical Activity* , 16(1), 44.

Chapter 18 :

- Mayo Clinic - Water: How much should you drink every day?

- Harvard T.H. Chan School of Public Health - The Nutrition Source: Water
- National Institute of Diabetes and Digestive and Kidney Diseases - Drinking Water and Health
- Environmental Protection Agency (EPA) - Water Quality Standards
- World Health Organization (WHO) - Drinking-water

Chapter 19 :

- American Academy of Nutrition and Dietetics. (2017). "Do You Need Supplements?"
- National Institutes of Health (NIH) Office of Dietary Supplements. (2021). "Vitamins and Minerals."
- The Environmental Working Group. (2020). "Sustainable Supplement Sourcing."
- Harvard T.H. Chan School of Public Health. (2020). "The Role of Supplements in a Healthy Diet."
- Nutrition and Food Science, "Plant-Based Supplements for Optimal Health," 2019.

Chapter 20 :

- "The Blue Zones: Lessons for Living Longer From the People Who've Lived the Longest" by Dan Buettner
- Harvard T.H. Chan School of Public Health, "The Nutrition Source: Healthy Eating Plate"
- World Health Organization (WHO), "Healthy Diet"
- "How Not to Die: Discover the Foods Scientifically Proven to Prevent and Reverse Disease" by Michael Greger
- American Heart Association, "Nutrition and Health"
- National Institute on Aging, "Eating and Aging"

- The American Journal of Clinical Nutrition, "Dietary Patterns and Long-Term Health"

Chapter 21 :
- "The Benefits of Eating Locally Sourced Foods." Environmental Protection Agency.
- "How to Encourage Children to Eat More Vegetables." Healthy Kids.
- "The Impact of Food Waste on the Environment." The Nature Conservancy.
- "Sustainable Eating: A Guide for Families." Environmental Working Group.
- "The Importance of Plant-Based Eating for the Environment." World Wildlife Fund (WWF).

Chapter 22 :
- FAO. (2018). *The State of Food and Agriculture 2018: Migration, Agriculture and Rural Development* . Food and Agriculture Organization of the United Nations.
- GRAIN. (2020). *Regenerative Agriculture and the Food Crisis: A Global Overview* . GRAIN.org.
- Beyond Meat. (2021). *Sustainability & Beyond* . Beyond Meat, Inc.
- Precision Agriculture for Development. (2019). *Precision Agriculture and Its Impact on Sustainable Farming Practices* . Precision Agriculture for Development.
- P. Smith, et al. (2020). *The Role of Technology in Reducing Food Waste* . Food Policy.

Made in the USA
Las Vegas, NV
10 April 2025